Keto Diet and Intermittent Fasting

for Beginners:

Keto diet and Intermittent Fasting for beginners: The Final Guide to Combining Ketogenic Diet and Intermittent Fasting for Fast Weight Loss for Women + 50 Recipes

Table of Content

Contents

Introduction

Obesity and the causes of being fat or obese. These are all tiny little problems that every person faces, yet they seem as if they are the most significant difficulties that one can cross at all. The reason for removing obesity is considered a lot challenging is because people lose their hope and determination. Hence, keto diet helps us a lot and is our choice to make. We can opt keto diet with intermittent fasting to enjoy the benefits.

You can dream and follow your dreams; if you look back, you can't move forward unless you learn. This is why obesity is increasing at a rate of 40% in the whole world. Women love sugar, and that is why their primary reason for obesity is sugar (diabetes), carbohydrates, trans fats, and not being physical at all (lazy – no physical activity). Even if your body does not show that it is obese, later it will, up to 25% of women become obese in their coming future.

The overweight or obesity affects many significant parts of the human body including, hormonal effects, biochemical changes, immunological physiology, metabolic malfunction, molecular physiology, diabetes, insulin resistance, even the tissue (adipose) accumulation rate malfunctions. Obesity causes risk of hyperglycemia. Hyperglycemia further causes many disasters and illness. They also cause cardiovascular diseases. This is also a major reason for the premature deaths in women worldwide.

The known risk factors: overconsumption of foods, sugary drinks, sodas, syrups are the source reason for illness in women leading to obesity.

You can overcome these severe problems just by intermittent fasting. It is not as if problems don't have their solutions. Solutions do exist. It depends on you if you are willing enough to convert your problem to your own advantage. Intermittent fasting is not as if you fast. You only schedule your eating habits. You only eat when the right time is there. You do not eat 24/7, that is the root of obesity. Constant snacking slacks you from your life. Not just your tasks, but also from your dreams. Follow a schedule and stick to it to maintain your body.

Once you achieve your goal, you will experience the benefits yourself. If you do not, you will live in a hell created by your brain forever. Individual guilt will glue to your mental stability. Hence you need to follow your dreams. If you do not like to go to the gym and thinks that it is difficult, remember, there is always another way. You can adopt intermittent fasting (90% rate approval by a survey).

Chapter 1: Introduction to ketogenic diet

When you are obese, trying to shape in your body or want to manage any health condition such as Type II Diabetes, then you may want to get rid of some extra pounds. There are various types of diets which are known and being practiced for rapid weight loss. Out of all the diets, the Ketogenic diet has gained massive popularity among people. A ketogenic diet is also known as "keto diet" is a renowned diet which is effective in rapid weight loss and in preventing from various health conditions such as coronary heart disease, Type II Diabetes, cancer and many others.

Before heading towards the details, let's have a look at the basics associated with the ketogenic diet. Our food comprises of fats, lipids, carbohydrates, vitamins, and proteins- which are essential for the optimal growth of an individual. Carbohydrates come in various forms and food items. The high concentration of carbs is present in dairy products like milk, ice cream, yogurt, eggs, fruits, and grains like rice, bread, cereals-legumes like beans- vegetables like potatoes and corn and dark chocolates. Proteins are abundant in animal foods such as milk, fish, eggs, yogurt, and chicken. Olives, nuts, beans, steak, chocolates, and dairy products are a rich source of fats.

Most of the people are the followers of low-fat, high-carb food pattern without knowing how it is adversely affecting their bodies and lives.

What is the ketogenic or keto diet?

Keto diet is a low-carb high-fat diet which enables the body to utilize fat as a fuel instead of producing glucose in the body. The body is forced to burn fat instead of carbohydrates in the body. Usually, the carbs in the food are converted into glucose and then are circulated the body. But in the ketogenic diet, there are fewer than 50 grams of carbohydrates which are taken up by the body, placing the body into a state of ketosis. When the body is in the state of ketosis, then it is encouraged to use fats instead of glucose to take out everyday activities.

It is understood that when we limit the intake of carbohydrates, then our body searches for an alternative as a fuel source. At that time, the body uses fat as an alternative fuel source. The body converts fat into glucose, which is then circulated throughout the body to perform everyday activities.

Due to a deficient supply of carbohydrates to the body, the liver converts fat into fatty acids and ketone bodies. The ketones and fatty acids are released into the bloodstream and are used as a source of energy.

The shifting of breakage of stored fats as fuel source happens when a body is getting fewer than 50 grams of carbohydrates for about two to four days. Keto diet is low in carbs and high in fats. The menu typically includes meat, vegetables, sausages, oil, fish, cheese, seeds, and much other protein and fat-enriched items. Because the diet is highly restrictive, only a few people can follow it for the long run.

What does low-carb, high fat mean in keto diet?

The low carb entails the presence of few carbohydrates, and high fat means the increased number of fats into the diet. The elevated level of fats in the diet pushes the body into a state of ketosis. The low level of carbohydrates forces the body to search for an alternative fuel source which is primarily the fat deposits in the body. Fat impacts less to the blood sugar levels as compared to the carbohydrates.

Keto Macros

Keto macro is the short form of keto macronutrients which include carbohydrates, fats, and proteins. The everyday intake of fats must be 70%, 25% of proteins and 5% of carbohydrates. In keto diet, it is essential to have an appropriate amount of macronutrients. Taking a balanced amount of micronutrients is necessary to get energy for everyday activities.

If you intend to lose weight, the total fat intake must be less than 60%. The exact amount of macronutrients is necessary for getting the best results of the diet. People pursuing a keto diet must not consume over 5% of carbohydrates daily.

Types of the ketogenic diet

Ketogenic diet comes with various types, which are as follows:

1) *Standard Ketogenic Diet (SKD)*

The standard ketogenic diet revolves around the high fat containing meals such as meat, butter, cheese, avocados, olives, fatty fish, eggs, nuts, and dark chocolates. Individual needs to intake 150 grams of fat per day to shift the metabolism from carbohydrates to fats. Not only this, but the person also needs to cut down the carbs rate from 300+ proteins to the 50 grams each day. Standard keto diet asks an individual to intake 90 grams of protein each day.

Macronutrients Ratio: 75% fats, 20% proteins and 5% carbohydrates

2) *Cyclical Ketogenic Diet (CKD)*

Cyclical keto is the one which comes with five days of the traditional keto diet and two non-keto days each week. This means you have to strictly follow the keto diet plan for five days and for the rest of two days you can go with whatever you want to. Some people who are pursuing this keto-diet save their two of non-keto days for special occasions such as marriages, birthdays, and vacations. For optimum results, an individual is asked to eat carbohydrate-rich foods on off days. It is indeed the best way to enjoy your dieting period.

Macronutrients ratio:

Keto days: 75% fats, 15-20% proteins, 5-10% carbohydrates

Non-keto days: 25%fats, 25%proteins, 50% carbohydrates

3) *Targeted Ketogenic Diet (TKD)*

An athlete-friendly diet which includes some more carbs than other forms of the keto diet. The diet is renowned among athletes who require some high level of carbs. About 20-30 grams of carbs are included in the diet of an individual so that person may be able to do high-intensity exercises. The person pursuing targeted keto diet can have dairy food, milk, and fruits into their diet. The additional carbs will not be stored into the body; instead, they will be burned off during exercise.

Macronutrients ratio: 65-70% fats, 20% proteins, 10-15% carbohydrates

4) *High-Protein Ketogenic Diet (HPKD)*

HPKD comes with a high ratio of protein intake. The follower of this plan needs to take 120 grams of protein along with 130 grams of fat each day. A large number of people of the keto diet are followers of this diet plan as it is comparatively easy to go with. Many nutritionists say that this plan may not result in the process of ketosis, but eventually, the HPKD aims at the weight loss of the person.

Macronutrients ratio: 60-65% fats, 30% proteins, 5-10% carbohydrates

Extensive research has been done on high protein and standard keto diets. The other two forms of keto diets (cyclical and targeted) are the advanced ones and are mostly practiced by athletes.

Basic Principles of Ketogenic Diet

While individual is going to select keto-diet type according to his personality and work type, then there are some basic principles which one needs to keep in mind.

- If you are a layman and want to follow a keto diet, then you must go for the Standard Keto Diet which includes 75% fats, 20% proteins, and 5% carbs.

- To make an accurate keto diet plan, you need to check the percentage of fat in your body.

- Add healthy fats in your diet plans such as olive oil, saturated fats, and Omega 3.

- A person who rarely does high-intensity exercise can pursue Standard keto Diet (SKD).

- If your carbohydrate level goes beyond 20 grams, then you should avoid low-carb containing food items.

- People who do high-intensity exercises regularly can go for Cyclical Keto Diet (CKD) and Targeted Keto Diet (TKD).

- People with the most advanced form of training or exercises can go for Cyclical Ketogenic Diet.

- People who crave to have snacks can take nuts, avocados, and coconut oil as an alternative.

- Standard Ketogenic Diet works best for the ones who pursue aerobic and endurance exercises such as running, biking, etc.

- If a person loses performance during exercise, then the best suitable diet plan for such person is TKD one.

- Being on the ketogenic diet, you don't need to check on the number of calories, go with what your body needs. Once you reach your weight loss goals, then you can have an eye on the calorie count.

- Bodybuilders and athletes can go for Cyclical Ketogenic Diet (CKD).

- Increase the water intake and drink 2 liters of water each day at least.

However, these guidelines are not strict about following. When people are going to figure out the appropriate type of ketogenic diet for them, then they can go for the ones which best fits in with their body needs. People are free to choose whatever best suits with them, but these guidelines will help them to be on singletrack.

One guideline which one strictly need to follow is that if a person is not onto high-intensity exercises daily, then he needs to stick with the Standard Ketogenic Diet (SKD) only.

Ketosis Symptoms

When the body of the person transitions into ketosis, the person experiences several symptoms known as the keto flu. The symptoms of keto flu include nausea, increased thirst, headache, and fatigue. These symptoms are the indication that your body is entering into ketosis while to ensure you can test the body ketone levels.

Testing for Ketosis

One can quantify the state of ketosis by performing breath, urine, and blood testing. The examination helps in checking whether the person has achieved the level of ketosis or not.

Three ways are typically done to test the ketosis within the human body:

- Blood testing
- Urine testing
- Breath testing

Blood testing

Testing blood can lead to the most accurate measurements of ketosis. The same procedure is used for the people undergoing diabetes to check their blood glucose levels. A blood BHB/glucose meter is used to measure blood glucose levels. Operating blood ketone meter is very easy and straightforward. All you need is to get a device, lancets, alcohol, lancet device, and test strips.

Taking a reading on blood ketone meter is very easy; you only have to keep these simple steps in mind:

- First and foremost thing to do is to remove the cap of your device and insert the lancets into it

- By rotating the lid of the invention, set your desired depth of puncture

- Next, arm the device until you hear the sound of the click

- Then place the strip into the reader

- Clean your left index fingertip with the sterile wipe and then put the finger firmly on the lancing device

- Squeeze the thumb to take out the drop of blood from it and then place your finger over strip (to make your blood absorb into it)

Wait until your reader gives you the results, and then you can analyze the results to check whether you have achieved the ketone levels or not.

Urine testing

Urine testing comes with various pros and cons. The examination is relatively inexpensive than blood testing yet not so accurate to be considered. There are multiple factors which affect urine testing and hence make it not so precise form of measurement. As we all are well aware that urine is a waste product, so on the ketone urine strip, the test will display what body is sweating out. This will not accurately indicate how much your body is using ketone. Not only this but with time, the body becomes adapted to ketones; therefore, through urine, there is a minimal amount of ketones which body sweats out. Others factors such as hydration can also lead to inconsistent results.

Breath testing

Breath testing devices are not so old, so they come with new technology in the market. The level of acetone is measured, which a body excretes out with the breath. As the type of testing is unique, therefore, there is minimal research done over it. Accuracy of the test has not been studied much; hence, the breath test is not considered as reliable as the blood testing.

Why is keto testing essential?

If you are the one pursuing keto diet, then checking out the ketone levels in the body is essential. It is necessary to know about the ketone levels for the ones who want to pursue a keto diet for weight loss or to combat with any medical condition. People having moderate ketone levels may need to add few ketone-level enhancing food items into their diets to reach the weight loss goals.

Some people take longer to enter into ketosis. Why?

There are various reasons people take longer to enter into the state of ketosis. Most of the time, people may unintentionally start taking an extra amount of carbs than recommended. An additional amount of carbs can stop producing ketone bodies, which is the ultimate way of placing the body into the state of ketosis. It is essential to take fewer carbs to enter into ketosis.

Another cause can be not taking a sufficient amount of fats on the keto diet. Generally, people are asked to intake 75% of fats every day to place their bodies into ketosis. When the prescribed amount of fats is not taken up by the individual, it deprives a person of entering into ketosis.

Intake of excess proteins can also make it difficult to enter into ketosis. A large number of proteins can make the body enter into the process of gluconeogenesis, which makes the body convert amino acids into glucose.

Other factors may include sleep, anxiety, stress, which makes it hard for the person to enter into ketosis.

Tips to get into ketosis rapidly

Getting into ketosis is not as easy as it seems to be. Having an appropriate amount of carbs proteins and fats are essential to achieve the state of ketosis.

- **Increase physical activity-** Enhanced physical activity will lead to more consumption of fats for fuel. Frequent exercise leads to the depletion of glycogen stores in the body, which eventually leads to the formation of ketone bodies.

- **Decrease carbs intake-** Decrease in carbs intake can more frequently lead to ketosis. The lower carb rate shifts the body mechanism towards the utilization of fats as a source of fuel. Taking 5 grams of carbs each day will help to achieve the ketosis goal.

- **Suppress appetite-** Eat less and eat healthily can lead to the ultimate ketosis goal. Nutritionists usually recommend fasting for short periods to achieve ketosis. If you crave to go out and have a meal, then you can pursue keto-friendly restaurants.

- **Intake high-quality fats-** In general, there is a prescription to intake 70-75% of healthy fats each day on a ketosis diet. Most of the day, the person needs to get in the avocados, coconut oil, nuts, meat, butter, eggs, and fatty acids.

- **Have a check on your snacks-** If a person craves to have meals, he must search for an alternative. Usually, when a person is traveling, it gets harder for a person to remain on keto-friendly foods. However, a person can take keto snacks with him to satisfy his cravings. Keto-friendly meals may include keto bars, keto nut butter, nuts, and seeds.

- **Test ketosis level regularly-** Testing ketone levels often helps the person to have an eye on whether the person is in the state of ketosis or not. Moreover, a person can schedule his keto diet plan according to the test results.

- **Take medium-chain triglyceride (MCT) supplement-** MCTs are known as the frequent fat absorbents which rapidly absorbs into the body. MCTs, help into the rapid conversion of fat into ketone bodies.

Get optimal results of the ketogenic diet

The keto diet revolves around the burning of fat cells to get fuel for the body. To get optimal results, the first and foremost thing which a person needs to keep in mind is to drink plenty of water. Keto diet encompasses the foods which make the person urge for the water. Therefore, a person pursuing a keto diet must drink enough water to stay away from dehydration.

Carbohydrates significantly hold the water concentration in the body, but when a person restricts carbohydrates, then water concentration starts to decline. Continuously measure your fat burn rate by testing the levels of ketosis to keep your body healthy. In keto diet always go for the secure food options which you can follow instead of sticking to the hard choices. The salads of various vegetables are an excellent option to remain in the state of ketosis.

Chapter 2: Importance of ketogenic diet

The ketogenic diet offers extraordinary benefits related to general health, weight loss, metabolic efficiency, and many others. Keto diet is the best way to lose your weight and get rid of many severe health conditions without having yourself starved.

When you adhere yourself with the defined set of eating habits, ketosis or fasting, then it can lead to rapid burning of fat cells of your body. Not only this, but keto diet helps in burning of glucose cells, which makes diet the choice of many.

There are a large number of health benefits which keto diet offers. Here are the few benefits which you will get on pursuing the ketogenic diet.

1) *Treating epilepsy*

Ketogenic diet brings epilepsy treatment option for people belonging to all age groups. First and foremost benefit, which makes the diet choice of many is its treatment of epilepsy. The ketogenic diet is widely known for controlling and treating seizures, along with many other positive health effects. The difficult-to-control disease can be controlled by following this simple diet.

How does it work?

During regular food days, the carbohydrates taken up by the body are converted into glucose and are then transported throughout the body. But with the keto diet, there are fewer than 50 grams of carbs which are taken up by the body. What happens when a person's intake of carbohydrates drops from 300 grams daily to 50 grams? During such conditions, the liver starts to burn fat of the body to fulfill the needs of the body.

The fat and fatty acids in the body are converted into ketone bodies. Those ketone bodies then go into the brain and replace glucose deposits there (ketones act as an energy source). Gradually when the number of ketone bodies increases in the blood, this puts the body into the state of ketosis. The high levels of ketones then function to reduce epileptic seizures.

The Research study results

Various research studies have been conducted to check the effect of the keto diet on the reduction of epileptic seizures. Half of the people following the keto diet have reported at least half of the decrease of their epileptic seizures.

Many researchers have claimed the keto diet to be more effective than many medicines for the treatment of seizures. Various research studies have recommended pursuing a keto diet to treat epilepsy if medications are not working.

a. Weight loss

A large number of people start following the keto diet due to its weight loss property. The diet is renowned for rapid weight loss with strict adherence to strict diet plans.

How does it work?

The brain of a person daily requires an appropriate amount of energy from a proper energy source to function optimally. Carbohydrates are burned by the liver to produce glucose, which is then circulated to the brain. When there is a lack of supply of carbohydrates for three to four days to the body, then the body searches for an alternative source of energy.

At that time, the body utilizes fat and burns it to produce ketone bodies. Ketone bodies can be used as an alternative to glucose in their absence. When the body starts to burn fat in the absence of sufficient carbs, then it results in rapid weight loss.

The research study results

Various research studies have been conducted to check the effect of the ketogenic diet on obese persons. The results have shown the significant impact of the keto diet over the reduction of body weight and BMI of participants.

Longitudinal research studies conducted on obese persons have not shown any significant side effects of the diet. Hence it is the beneficial type of diet to pursue long run.

b. Minimizes heart diseases by improving cholesterol levels

Lower carbohydrate-containing diets are said to be ideal for the reduction of high cholesterol levels and consequently the heart diseases. The leading cause of coronary heart diseases is the elevated LDL (bad) cholesterol level in the body.

How does it work?

The frequent intake of healthy fats during keto diet can lead to the improved HDL (good) cholesterol levels in the body. The diet significantly decreases the LDL (bad) cholesterol levels in the body. This consequently leads to the reduction of heart diseases in the people.

The diet keeps the person away from the intake of LDL cholesterol, enhancing food items. The consumption of LDL cholesterol levels inhibiting food items keeps the person at low risk from heart issues.

The research study results

A research study conducted showed that keto diet could lead to a significant decrease in LDL cholesterol and an increase in HDL (good) cholesterol.

Another research study was conducted on women; the results showed that there was significant decrease in LDL cholesterol levels, which lead to lower cardiovascular disease risk in females.

c.   *Treats women with Polycystic Ovarian Syndrome (PCOS)*

A rapidly growing issue within females is the Polycystic Ovarian Syndrome (PCOS). The syndromes result in the enlargement of ovaries and produce cysts within. High-carbohydrate diet may enhance the PCOS. PCOS greatly influences fertility and is said to be responsible for over 70% of infertility problems within females. The main reason behind the syndrome is elevated levels of insulin, which makes the ovaries to produce androgens and inhibits the production of sex hormone i.e., globulin.

When there is the high production of androgen and lower secretion of globulin, the testosterones start to float into the blood and influence many body cells. This results in many health conditions such as mood swings, fatigues, aggression, increase in hair production on the body, infertility, and many other symptoms.

How does it work?

The decrease in weight due to the keto diet can lead to decreased symptoms of PCOS. The reduction in insulin levels is associated with the reduction in symptoms of PCOS.

The research study results

There is a minimal number of research studies conducted on to check the impact of a keto diet on the PCOS. However, one pilot study was conducted, which showed that women who were following the keto diet had a significant loss in their weight. Not only have this, but the number of free-floating testosterone also decreased significantly.

Moreover, the fasting insulin levels, which were greatly responsible for the syndrome, dropped significantly. Despite, the women in the research study were declared as the infertile ones got pregnant after pursuing the keto diet. More research is needed to be done on the following issue to get better results.

d. Overcoming Type-II Diabetes

When the blood sugar or blood glucose level rise beyond the average level, then this results in the Type-II Diabetes. Type-II Diabetes encompasses higher levels of glucose, which can cause a person to undergo serious health issues. The keto diet is said to overcome the Type-II Diabetes to a greater extent.

How does it work?

Carbohydrates are the great source of glucose as it converts into the glucose to be rotated around the brain. Therefore, with the keto diet when there are low carbs levels, then there will automatically decrease in the levels of glucose. This will help in the control of Type-II Diabetes, which causes due to the high level of blood glucose.

The research study results

Various research studies have been conducted to check the impact of keto diet over the control of Type-II Diabetes. One research study found that low-carbohydrate containing food can significantly lead to controlled blood sugar levels in type II Diabetics. The low consumption of carbohydrates also improves the blood sugar levels to the average level. People who want to control their type II Diabetes can go for the keto diet, which significantly controls the health condition.

e. Minimizes Alzheimer's disease

Intake of too much carbohydrate can lead to the formation of plaque in the brain and hence impairs the brain functioning. High-carbohydrate intake can reduce the cognitive abilities of the person. Not only this, but the memory of the person also gets affected adversely. Therefore, consumption of carbohydrates for patients with Alzheimer's disease is also prohibited.

How does it work?

Ketogenic diet comes with a low level of carbohydrates, which is the plus point for the patients of Alzheimer's disease. People with Alzheimer's disease are asked to lower their carbohydrate intake to reverse the disease.

The research study results

Different experiments and research studies on the ketogenic diet have found that ketone bodies can enhance the memory functioning of people undergoing Alzheimer's disease. Various tests were also conducted where subjects were given with the oil which was responsible for enhancing the ketone levels in the body. The results of the experiments have shown that Alzheimer's patients have shown a significant change in their memory. The memory recall of the patients was substantially enhanced.

f. Helps to reduce cancer risk

The ketogenic diet is considered to be having the potential for combating with cancer. The ketogenic diet is said to be an alternative therapy for the treatment of cancer patients.

How does it work?

Keto diet is investigated to be the one to reduce the risk of cancer. When the keto diet is given with conventional treatment, it results in the significant improvement in the condition of patients. The primary source for cancer cells is glucose, due to keto diet cancer cells get deprived of the glucose, which leads to the death of cancer cells. The cancer cells in keto diet can no longer get their fuel-which they get from the glucose.

Secondly, the keto diet is responsible for the suppression of insulin growth factor. The critical factor in the progression of cancer cells is insulin growth. Carbohydrates enhance the level of insulin growth factor. Hence the low level of carbohydrates can lead to the suppression of insulin growth factor, which frequently increases the cancer cells level.

The research study results

The research studies done on cancer patients have shown a significant improvement in the condition of most of the patients. Some patients showed complete remission, whereas some experienced progression in the situation once they stopped the diet.

g. Reduces Migraines

Interestingly, the ketogenic diet has seen to reduce severe migraines. Following keto diet can lead to the reduction of intensity and frequency of the migraine attacks.

How does it work?

The high level of ketones in a keto diet can lead to the inhibition of inflammation within the brain cells of the person. The food also enhances the functioning of mitochondrial brain metabolism, which helps in the reduction of severe migraine. High ketone levels are also responsible for the reduction of oxidative stress. The ketones also block the high concentrations of glutamate.

How ketogenic diet is beneficial in general?

Keto diets help deal with specific conditions, but there are some benefits which everyone experiences. Here are some of the ketogenic diets which everyone experiences.

1) Enhances energy

The keto diet improves the mitochondrial function, which provides more power to the body cells. Keto diet produces less reactive oxygen species, which also elevates the energy level of the person. Ketogenic diet keeps the person active throughout the day and performs his activities while being with full of energy.

2) Appetite Control

The most significant benefit of the diet is that it controls the appetite of the person. The person pursuing a keto diet does not feel hungry often and stays away from unnecessary cravings, which make a person engage in bad eating habits. Many people want to control their appetite to keep their physique in a track.

3) *Improves brain functioning*

The game-changer diet enhances the brain functioning of the person. Keto diet makes the brain cells work more efficiently. The brain inflammation also reduces, which leads to the increased activity of the brain. The person following the keto diet plan can perform cognitively better. High level of glutamate and a little level of GABA can lead to a lack of concentration.

The keto diet balances the levels of GABA and glutamate so that the person can fully concentrate or pay attention to his activities. The brain is the fattiest part of the body requires high-fat levels to function optimally. As keto diet is enriched in fat, it leads to better brain functioning.

4) *Reduces stress and anxiety*

The enhancement in the production of GABA helps in the reduction of stress and anxiety of person, thus making the person calm and relax. The low levels of sugar and fats can also lead to a reduced level of stress and anxiety. A research study conducted on mice in this regard has indicated that mice showed a reduced level of anxiety.

5) *Enhances body composition*

Ketogenic is the more significant source of weight loss but many people who want to pursue a keto diet do not want to lose weight; what should they do? The keto diet although may be responsible for weight loss, but it also increases the muscle mass.

6) *Sleep better*

People often come with the problem that they had difficulty in falling asleep. Some come with the issue that if they get to sleep, they cannot sleep deeper. With the keto diet, the person may get sound and deeper sleep. During the adjustment phase, people may have insomnia: however, once people fully adjust to the ketosis, they can sleep sounder and more in-depth. The diet helps in making a person feel relaxed and rested.

7) *Reduces inflammation*

Inflammation is often said to be due to heart problems, high glucose levels, arthritis, or any other health condition. As nutritional ketosis is linked with the reduction of all these conditions, then it directly or indirectly reduces the inflammation as well. The inflammation level in the body is measured by conducting various blood tests on the patient.

The ketone bodies produce few radicals and switches off inflammatory pathways. This is advantageous because chronic inflammation can lead to chronic diseases such as heart diseases or cancers. Another benefit of the ketosis is that it may not only decrease the inflammation but can reduce the pain as well.

8) *Improves stamina*

The endurance level of the person increases with the keto diet. The physical strength of the person rises as he utilizes the stored fat to stay active. We all are well aware that carbs can melt quickly than fats. Therefore, fats can last longer than carbs, and hence, the keto diet keeps the person active. The body and mind continuously get energy through fat storage, which enables the person to exercise for a longer time.

Hence people, whose body is on fat, will have higher endurance than the ones whose body is on carbs.

9) *Prevents aging*

Histone Deacetylase is an enzyme which prevents the functioning of the Metallothionein 2A and Forkhead box O3. However, when there is a need to avoid the stress, then Histone Deacetylase activates both the genes to prevent the body from the oxidative stress. Moreover, the low blood sugar levels prevent the person from aging, which is the best thing about the ketogenic diet.

10) *Vanishes acne*

Many people who are on a keto diet have reported a significant decrease in their acne after they started having a keto diet. The most frequent cause of acne is insulin. The keto diet results in a low level of blood sugar into the body, which means the insulin level is much reduced in the body. Thus low levels of insulin lead to the reduction of acne.

Chapter 3: Things to eat and avoid on keto diet

When it comes to losing weight, dealing with any severe health condition or it's the matter of healthy living, then following a proper plan on the keto diet is essential. Keto diet is a hard-to-follow plan which can be followed by a minimal number of people for the long run. Keto diet limits the person to healthy eating by eliminating all the junks and high-carb foods. A rule of thumb for keto is to eat healthy, fresh, and real food. Here are the fruits, vegetables and food items which you need to eat during your keto journey:

Fruits

Usually, the conception associated with the fruits is that they are high in carbs and hence are not recommended on the keto diet, which is wrong. Fruits are indeed high on carbs, but there are fruits which do not have high glucose or carbs levels, so they must be taken up by the person on the keto diet. Some fruits come with the more top water level, and deficient carbs levels- these fruits are said to be keto-friendly fruits.

1. *Raspberries*

Raspberries are one of the keto-friendly fruits which have low carb levels. The high levels of antioxidants make the fruit friendly for a healthy body. Raspberries are recommended to pursue as they come with a deficient level of sugar, which is a plus point for keto diet followers. Eating raspberries can enhance the health of your heart. The fruit is renowned for promoting the health of the heart and for preventing high blood pressures and heart diseases.

2. *Grapefruit*

Grapefruit is full of Vitamin C, potassium, and fiber is known as the best option for weight loss. The additional body fat can be burnt with the glass of juice of grapefruit. Have a glass full of grapefruit juice daily and shed some extra pounds.

3. *Avocadoes*

Avocadoes are renowned for the least carbohydrate content. Not only this, avocadoes provides the person with the healthy monosaturated fats which are known a life changer for the people with heart issues.

4. Peaches

Peaches are less sweet and have a shallow content of carbohydrates. You can have peach in the form of juice or can take up with cottage cheese to reach your diet goals.

5. Strawberries

Strawberries are known for their deliciousness, sweet, and mouth-watering taste. In keto diet, the berries can be taken in the raw form, or you can add it in your fruit salad. Moreover, you can blend them to make mouth-watering smoothie for yourself. The strawberry smoothie is not only good for your skin but also has antioxidant and anti-inflammatory properties. The fruit is keto-friendly making it the choice of many.

6. Watermelon

Watermelon is the fruit available in summers and is enriched with water. The high concentration of water makes the fruit low on carbs and hence is the best fruit to have in your keto diet. You can use watermelon in raw form or can add it in a salad or can have a delicious smoothie. The fruit keeps the person hydrated, which best goes with the demands of the keto diet.

Vegetables

During the keto diet, where there is a limited number of carbs, then vegetables work best there. Vegetables are a great source of nutrition and are lower in calories, which make them a big YES on the keto diet. Here are some vegetables with the lowest-carb rate.

1. *Cauliflower*

Cauliflower is renowned for patients of cancer. The vegetable is rich in Vitamin C, Phytonutrients, and folate, which make it a must-to-have in diet vegetable. To get rid of fat, you can take in the raw cauliflower. Otherwise, you can roast the cauliflower a little and can intake to get optimal results.

2. *Spinach*

Salads are the best thing to have during your diet. When it comes to spinach, it is deficient on carb rate. Therefore, to have the spinach salad is the best thing to achieve your diet goals. You can take spinach salad with chicken or strawberries.

3. Cucumbers

Cucumbers are rich in water concentration and are very refreshing to have in salads. You can have cucumber in your salads regularly as the high level of water makes the lower carbohydrates levels in the vegetable. You can have them with peel or without them but preferred is to have them without skin. They not only help you in your keto diet but also fulfill the water needs of the body.

4. White mushrooms

White mushrooms are also low in carbs and can be ideal to have in breakfast. You can add them to the omelet with egg white to get low-carb breakfast.

5. Tomatoes

Tomatoes are widely known for their benefits and are taken up by the keto-diet followers. The person following the keto diet can take tomatoes in raw form, can roast them. Moreover, a person can add tomatoes into the salads for better use. Tomatoes taste good and can prevent the person from various strokes.

6. *Lemon*

Lemon is known for antioxidant properties and helps to fight with free radicals. You can take a glass full of water and squeeze one lemon into it and can make it. It helps in healthy digestion.

7. *Broccoli*

Broccoli includes the cabbages and radishes. Various research studies have shown that broccoli helps in the reduction of insulin resistance, which prevents type II diabetes. Not only it is helpful in the prevention of Type II diabetes, but it also prevents cancer.

8. *Garlic*

Garlic is known for enhancing immune function. It is known as a good source of weight loss and resists the common cold. Garlic is beneficial in decreasing blood pressure.

9. Celery

Celery has deficient levels of carbohydrates. The vegetable is an excellent source of vitamin K and has antioxidant properties which prevent and treats cancer.

10. Onions

Onions are known for the reduction of LDL cholesterol levels. The high antioxidant properties help in lowering the blood pressure of the person. Onion is useful for the treatment of overweight and to treat Polycystic Ovary Syndrome (PCOS) in females.

Other foods

1. Egg white

The best thing to add in your diet plan is egg white. Egg white is considered best for those who want to lose their weight or belly fat. Eggs are also lower in carbs and proteins rate. Eggs enhance the hormones which make the person feel full and balance the blood sugar levels. Consumption of egg whites can save you from many health issues.

To consume them, boil the egg and separate egg white and yellow. The yellow part holds a lot of cholesterol, which is not keto-friendly. You can make the omelet of egg white to get rid of the belly fat. Hence add it in your everyday diet plan to get the best results.

2. *Yogurt*

The high concentration of calcium is essential for the prevention of fat cells. Yogurt is the rich source of calcium, which reduces obesity, high blood pressure, and minimizes the high cholesterol levels. Yogurt is an all-rounder as it helps you in your weight loss and supports your immune system.

3. *Cheese*

Cheese attracts a lot number of people due to being delicious. Although cheese has a high level of saturated fat, it does not contribute to cardiac issues. Having cheese daily and prevent loss of muscle mass and signs of aging. The low carb and high-fat ratio make it keto-friendly.

4. *Meat*

Meat is renowned for low carb rates. Meat is enriched in vitamin B, Potassium, Zinc, and Selenium. Being rich in high-quality protein and low-carb rate makes it friendly to have on a keto diet.

5. *Coconut oil*

The properties of coconut oil make it go best with the keto diet principles. Coconut oil helps in increasing the ketone bodies. The patients who have Alzheimer's disease, cancer, or any nervous system issue can increase the intake of coconut oil. As coconut oils are a mix of medium-chain triglycerides (MCTs), they are beneficial in the formation of ketones and are a great source of energy.

6. *Butter*

To add on fats in the diet, enhance your butter intake. Butter has deficient levels of carbohydrates whereas high levels of fats which go best with the keto diet. Many people believe that butter contributes to the heat issues, but it has seen that saturated fat is not responsible for heart diseases.

List of the keto diet foods

Foods to Eat

Dairy Products

Dairy products, in combination with meats, are used in ketogenic diet to get optimal results. In the ketogenic diet, a large portion of your food must be comprised of fats and oils, vegetables, fruits, and proteins.

Dairy products which are processed are not prescribed as they are high on the number of carbohydrates. While going for dairy products, choose the ones which are high in fats but low on carbs. Many people have allergies to lactose; therefore; they must stick with the long-aged dairy products.

You can have sauces from the dairy products to add some extra fats into your meal. Always keep in mind that dairy products come with the proteins as well.

Here are the dairy products which you need to have in your keto diet:

- **Heavy whipping cream-** you can use it on salads while on the keto diet.

- **Butter and ghee-** butter is almost 80% fat whereas ghee is 100% fat. You can go for them both.

- **Butter-** butter is responsible for giving ghee the nutty taste. You can have it on your keto diet.

- **Yogurt-** yogurt has its utmost benefits; you can add it into your keto diet.

Fats and oils

Get fats from natural sources such as nuts and butter. Take the high amount of fats to set in the process of ketosis in the body. Majority of the food which a person intakes while on keto diet comprises of high fats. While having fats, keep your choices in mind as you are free to have fats in your diet. A large number of lipids in the keto diet makes the person choose the items according to his choice as he can select from a large number of items.

Fats are an essential part of the body, but they can be dangerous as well because there are many fatal types of fats which one must avoid.

To get the appropriate kind of fats, one must need to have extensive knowledge about the fats. Unhealthy fats must be avoided in the keto diet to get the optimal results of the diet. Fats come in numerous types, some of which are as follows:

- **Trans Fats-** Trans fats are processed ones; therefore, they must be avoided altogether. The processes food comprises of chemicals. The keto diet makes sure that a person does not take any chemical containing food item. Therefore, trans fats are a big NO in the keto diet. Trans fats are considered to be linked with many health conditions such as cardiac issues, high blood pressures, and many others.

- **Monounsaturated Fats-** These fats are a big YES on the keto diet. One can take these fats. Some of the examples of monounsaturated fats are nuts, avocados, sunflower oil, and peanut oil.

- **Saturated Fats-** Saturated fats contain fat animal products, and one can intake the food items containing saturated fats. These fats include cream, cheese, fatty meats, coconut oil, kernel oil, and butter.

- **Polyunsaturated Fats-** the frozen polyunsaturated fats are not good and must be avoided, whereas fresh can be taken on the keto diet. These fats include olives, olive oil, avocados, avocado oil, nuts, fatty fish, and seeds.

Highly prescribed forms of fats are the saturated and monounsaturated ones because they are chemically stable and are have less inflammatory tendencies. While taking fish, always keep the balanced amount to balance between the Omega3 and Omega6. People who do not like fish can go for fish oil.

Nuts and seeds can be high in inflammatory omega6; therefore, take the appropriate amount of peanuts, almonds, sunflower oil, and walnuts. To keep Omega3 and 6 in normal ranges, eat fatty fish, take minimum snacks, and have fewer dessert items. As Omega3 and Omega6 are essential to the body but the excess of anything can be dangerous.

Here are the items high on fats and oils and you need to have in your diet:

- Avocados

- Nuts

- Walnuts

- Butter

- Peanuts

- Cheese

- Avocado oil

- Fatty fish

- Fish oil

- Coconut oils

- Egg yolks

Non-starchy Vegetables

Always go for the above-ground vegetables, which are leafy and green. You can take the frozen or fresh vegetables both. Although vegetables are of more significant benefit in the healthy ketogenic diet but selecting the appropriate vegetables is essential.

The vegetables which are nutrients enriched and contain low levels of carbs must be consumed in the keto diet. The dark and leafy vegetables are asked to take on a keto diet. You can go for both frozen and fresh vegetables as both have an equal amount of nutrients.

The vegetables grown below the ground must be avoided because they may contain a high rate of carbs. However, a moderate amount of underground vegetables can be consumed. Always check out the number of macronutrients that different vegetables hold.

Vegetables such as lettuce, spinach, cucumber, bacilli, celery, radishes, and spaghetti squash must be added into the diet. Underground vegetables have a high level of carbohydrates; therefore, they must be avoided. You must avoid:

- **Starchy vegetables-** altogether avoid starch-rich vegetables such as potatoes, etc

- **High carb vegetables-** beetroots, corn, sweet potatoes.

Protein

Meat is a good source of proteins. The meat which comes from the animals who were grass-fed and pasture-raised prevents the person from the attack of bacteria. Darker meat is always a good option than white meat. Fatty fish is a good source of Omega3. One thing which you need to keep in mind is that too much protein intake does not go with the keto diet.

Unprocessed meats must be preferred. Try to have a moderate amount of meats as they are high in proteins which do not come under the keto diet. Therefore, always go for the average amount of meat.

Too high levels of protein can lead to the lower production of ketone bodies and hence increases the blood glucose level. So, intake of protein under the prescribed amount is always the best option. You can balance the protein level by taking sauces. You can also pair your protein foods with fattier dishes or items such as protein to create a balance. It is always essential to intake a moderate level of protein.

To get protein and high levels of fats at the same time, you can go for the meat of lamb. The meat of lamb contains high fats and sufficient amount of proteins. Here are some protein-enriched food items you need to add into your ketogenic diet:

- **Beef-** cooked beef, steak.
- **Poultry-** chicken, hen, duck, pheasant, and many other wild animals.

- **Nuts-** natural, unsweetened nuts, legumes high on Omega 6, almond butter for the excess of fats. While consuming legumes, be careful that you may not get a higher concentration of legumes.

- **Fish-** Rainbow trout, herring, and tuna, wild-caught salmon, catfish, mahi-mahi and others. Try to go for the fat-enriched fishes.

- **Sausages-** go for the sausages which contain a low rate of carbs and the higher concentration of fats. Try to avoid the nitrates level.

- **Eggs-** you can have boiled fried, half-boiled, high fried.

Nuts and Seeds

Nuts are beneficial in a keto diet but to a limited extent. Taking the high number of nuts, especially peanuts, can result in inflammation within the body of the person. Raw nuts are used as the garnishing of meals and to give them texture and flavors. Many of the people use nuts as snacks, which provides very health-related benefits.

Nuts are fat-enriched items but don't forget that they have carbohydrate counts as well. Therefore, take the nuts to the moderate level. Nuts are high in Omega 6 fatty acids, which is another reason you must be careful while taking in the nuts.

Nuts are available in various categories such as some come with low carbohydrate levels, whereas some have high carbohydrate count while others have a moderate count. You must need to choose the ones which best goes with your keto diet plan. Here are the various types, from which you need to select the one which best goes with the keto diet:

- **Low carb nuts**- Best types of nuts to you need to pursue are with the low carbohydrate counts. The healthy nuts that are low in carbs are walnuts, hazelnuts, almonds, brazil nuts, and pecans.

- **High carb nuts**- High carb nuts are highly prohibited on the keto diet. Pistachios, cashews are examples of high carb-containing nuts.

- **Moderate carb nuts**- Peanuts, pine nuts contain an average level of carb; therefore they must be taken very rarely.

People often use nut and seed flour as an alternative to regular flour when they are on a keto diet. People on the keto diet also use seed and nut flour on for the baking and dessert recipes. It has been seen that combining flour for the baking purpose has a meager count of carbohydrates.

While combining flours, you also need to keep in mind the proportion of various nuts. Sometimes, the combination of flours can lead to a large number of carbs. Therefore, be careful while combining your flours for baking purposes.

Sugar addictions

A large number of people have severe sugar addictions, which can affect the keto diet of the person. People who are sugar enthusiast stay on a keto diet with very difficulty. Consumption of sugar can lead to the secretion of dopamine, which leads to the addiction. With continuous use of sugar, a person gets addicted and hence craves for the sugar.

When on the keto diet, your body struggles to shift from high carb to ketogenic diet, and then the cravings get in and try to prevent the person from going towards the diet plan. The desire of the person gets so intense that the person may want to quit the keto diet.

Not only for sugar, but the body of the person also craves for the foods which lack in nutrients. You can fulfill the craving of these foods by taking in alternative food. Such as instead of chocolate you can go for nuts and seeds, instead of oily foods you can have cheese, and spinach.

Sauces

For sauces lover, there may be a grey side on a keto diet as the diet does not allow the person to take in the pre-made sauces and spices. Already made sauces and condiments come up with sweeteners which are not keto-friendly.

If you want to have sauces and can't live without them, then you can make ones for yourself at your place. Make sauces by adding the ingredients which come under the keto diet. Keep your hand light on high carbs and go with a little watery sauce. Hollandaise and brown butter sauces are the keto-friendly ones.

When you need sauces in every condition, and then make ones for your self. Always check the number of ingredients and nutrition you are adding in the condiments and keep in mind whether the sauce you are making is following your keto diet plan or not.

The pre-made sauces which you need to avoid includes:

- Ketchup

- Mayonnaise

- Salad dressing

- Barbecue sauce

- Horseradish sauce

- Worcestershire sauce

- Flavored syrups

Spices

Monitoring spices on the keto diet is very crucial because even a small amount of spices can add up to the carbs count. Sauces are the most favorite part of people to add on any mean, but they are highly

prohibited on a keto diet.

When it comes to spices, they come in sufficient carb levels. Spices

can enhance the carb level, so make sure to keep a light hand while

adding them. Spices enthusiasts can look for the alternatives available

for spices such as sea salt can be used instead of table salt. Pre-made

spices come with the sugar added in them; therefore, avoid such spices

as much as you can.

Regular usage of spices is okay because spices contain a reasonable

amount of carbs but using a large number of spices can be alarming.

Here is the list of herbs and spices you can use on the keto diet:

- Tarragon

- Mint

- Basil

- Black pepper

- Cloves

- Coriander

- Garam masala

- Parsley

- Thyme

Foods to Avoid

Keto diet is a hard-to-follow diet. The diet comes with various restrictions and gives the followers an adamant time to get to their goals. Figuring out which foods you need to limit is very challenging. Daily carbs target helps the person to choose the foods which he needs to go with and to avoid the ones which are not suitable for him. It is always better to go for natural and fresh foods than the processed and frozen ones. Here are some of the foods you need to limit to get to your ketogenic diet goals:

- **Fruits-** Bananas, dates, pear, and mangoes are carbohydrate-rich foods which need to be avoided on the keto diet.

- **Starchy vegetables-** Many vegetables come with high fiber rate, which can lead to excessive weight gain or high blood sugar levels. High-starch vegetables come with the high levels of carbs which must be avoided to reach the ultimate keto diet goals. These vegetables include sweet potatoes, corns, and beets.

- **Low-fat foods-** Low-fat foods tend to bear high carbs rate because they come up with high levels of sugar.

- **Sweetened yogurt-** Plain yogurt is essential in keto diet but doesn't mix it with sweetened yogurt as it is just the opposite. Sweetened yogurt comes with high sugar levels, which makes it unfriendly for the keto diet.

- **Grains-** Grains such as pasta, cereal, rice, wheat, and barley much be avoided. These grains contain very high levels of carbs, which works just opposite to the keto diet.

- **Juices-** Try to avoid juices, although they are enriched with nutrients they contain high carbs levels. Fruit juices are very high in carbs, so say a big NO to fruit juices on the keto diet. Vegetable juices are low on carbs than fruit juices, but still, they contain sufficient carbs which are not good on a ketogenic diet.

- **Beans-** Beans are high in fiber, but they come with a fair amount of carbohydrates. Avoid lentils, chickpeas, pinto beans, peas, and black beans.

Chapter 4: Keto diet recipes

Keto breakfast recipes

A joyful and wishful breakfast makes the whole day go by pleasant and happier. A wishful breakfast for many may encompass the syrupy plate of pancakes which has carb rush. If you are a keto diet follower, then you may need to be very selective while looking for your breakfast. You have to avoid many sugar and carb-rich recipes. Here are the breakfast recipes which are the best ones to pursue a ketogenic diet. All the recipes are lower on carb levels. These keto-friendly breakfast recipes will keep you satisfied all your day.

1. Keto-friendly egg muffins

The recipe requires very little time to prepare and hence is time-saving. Egg muffins are all you need to satisfy your appetite as it is delicious, easy to make, and perfect for your keto-friendly breakfast.

Ingredients

- Eggs- 12

- Cooked bacon or chopped air-dried chorizo or salami- 5 ounce

- Green or red pesto- 2 tbsp

- Cheese (shredded)- 6 ounce

- Scallions (finely chopped)- 2

- Salt and pepper (according to taste)

Directions

- Take out eggs; add red or green pesto, salt, and pepper. Whisk it well.

- Add your favorite cheese and again stir the eggs.

- Take muffin tin with insertable, non-stick baking cups. You can grease your muffin tin with the butter.

- Now add chorizo and scallions at the bottom of the muffin tin.

- Preheat the oven for (175°C) or 350°F.

- Pour the batter of eggs over the scallions and chorizo in the muffin tin

- Bake muffins for almost 15-20 minutes. You can vary the time of the baking according to the size of your muffin cups.

Note: You can serve muffins to six persons. These muffins are what you need for your keto diet. Your children may love the recipe. You can store the egg muffins into the refrigerator for 3-4 days.

2. *Chia Pudding*

Being a pudding lover and pursuing keto-diet can put you to a challenging situation. But we have a solution for your pudding cravings. The blend of Chia seeds and coconut milk can give you a keto-friendly pudding. The pudding comes with the high number of Omega 3 and hence has anti-inflammatory tendencies. Easy to make and is less time taking. You can mix all the ingredients the night before, and the next day you can have it in breakfast.

Ingredients

- Chia seeds- ¼ cup
- Full-fat coconut milk- 1 cup
- Honey ½ teaspoon

Directions

- Take a small bowl or Mason jar. Mix all the ingredients, i.e., coconut milk, chia seeds, and honey well.

- Refrigerate it overnight.

- In breakfast, remove the pudding and make sure that it looks thick.

- You can top the budding with keto-friendly fruits and nuts.

- Enjoy the fresh and healthy pudding.

Note: make sure that pudding is thick; otherwise you may not get desired taste.

3. Eggs and Bacon

Although bacon is processed meat and is considered unhealthy, it has the great qualities which go fit with the keto diet. Bacon has a meager carb ratio, which makes it friendly on the keto diet. To add variation in your keto breakfast recipe, you can have this recipe once or twice a week.

Ingredients

- Bacon

- Eggs- 4

- Spices- to taste (optional)

Directions

- Take a pan and place bacon over it to fry.

- Beat 4 eggs into the bowl and then fry them in the bacon fat.

- To add some flavor, add salt, pepper, onion or garlic powder to taste.

- Once fried, place the egg into bacon. Enjoy healthy, keto-friendly breakfast.

Note: do not over fry the bacon or egg. Sprinkle spices over the egg while frying. Keep the proportion of spices in mind.

Keto lunch recipes

Making a delicious and keto-friendly lunch has been very easy with our guide. Here are the incredible ideas for your keto-friendly lunchtime.

1. Keto-friendly meat pie

Everyone loves cheese, and hence this recipe is the best one for the ones who want cheese topped cake in their lunch box. The method is easy-to-follow and all you want to have at your lunchtime.

Ingredients

For crust

- Coconut flour- 4tbsp

- Sesame seeds- 4tbsp

- Almond flour- ¾ cup

- Olive or coconut oil- 3 tbsp

- Egg- 1

- Water- 4 tbsp

- Salt- to taste

For filling

- Cheese- 7 oz. (shredded)

- Cottage cheese- 8 oz.

- Tomato paste- 4 tbsp

- Salt and pepper- to taste

- Ground beef- 20 oz.

- Yellow onion- ½ (chopped)

- Garlic clove- 1(chopped)

Directions

- Fry finely chopped onion and garlic in olive oil until onion gets soft. Add beef meat and keep on frying. After a few minutes add oregano or basil, salt, and pepper.

- Lower the heat and add tomato paste and then let it simmer for 15-20 minutes. During this time, make dough for the crust.

- Make the dough in the food processor by adding all the dough ingredients. You can make dough with your hands as well.

- Take deep-dish pie pan and place parchment paper in it. Before placing paper, grease the pan well. Spread the dough in the pan with the help of your hands. Prick the dough with the fork.

- Place the pan into the preheated oven (175°C), and pre-bake the crust for around 15 minutes. Once the crust is baked, remove it and add meat in it and layer shredded and cottage cheese over it.

- Bake it on lover rack for 30-35 minutes or until when your pie turns into golden color.

Note: you can store keto meat pie for 4 days into the fridge and for 2-3 months into the freezer.

2. Keto lunch salad

Being a salad lover and on the keto diet can bring you good news. As in keto, you can have a variety of salads. One of the salads here is mouthwatering and handy as well. You can have it in your lunch.

Ingredients

- Smoked salmon or chicken- 4 oz.

- Leafy greens- 1 oz.

- Red bell peppers- 1 oz.

- Cucumber- 1 oz.

- Scallion- ½

- Cherry tomatoes- 1 oz.

- Mayonnaise- ¼ cup

Directions

- Finely chop all the vegetables. Take a jar and put any of the dark leafy vegetable of your choice at the bottom. You can take lettuce, spinach or arugula.

- Add all the vegetables including onion rings, chopped carrot and bell peppers, avocados and tomatoes in layers.

- Top the salad with smoked salmon or grilled chicken. Moreover, you can top it with boiled egg whites or tuna fish. Olives, nuts, and cheese can also be added for additional flavor.

- You can add a little amount of mayonnaise for the dressing.

Note: Add a little amount of mayonnaise to stay under the keto diet.

3. Salmon keto burgers

Salmon and burger lovers can satisfy their appetites with these salmon burgers while being on the keto diet. They are comfortable and straightforward to make. You can have salmon burgers with green mash and lemon butter for additional taste.

Ingredients

For Salmon burgers

- Salt- to taste

- Salmon- 1 ½ lbs

- Yellow onion- ½

- Egg- 1

- Pepper- to taste

- Butter or olive oil- 2 oz.

For lemon butter

- Butter- 4 oz.

- Lemon juice- 2 tbsp

- Salt and pepper- to taste

For green mash

- Broccoli- 1lb

- Butter- 5 oz.

- Parmesan cheese- 2 oz.

- Salt and pepper- to taste

Directions

- Add all the ingredients along with salmon fish into the food processor. Pulse the ingredients for 40-50 seconds until you get a coarse mixture.

- Shape 5-6 burgers and fry until they become little brown from both sides.

- Trim the broccoli and chop it well into small pieces.

- Take a pot and add water and salt into it and bring it to boil. Once the water starts boiling add broccoli into it and cooks until broccoli becomes soft. Drain the broccoli.

- Now mix broccoli with other mixture with the help of a blender. Mix butter and parmesan cheese as well.

- Make lemon butter and green mash by mixing all the ingredients.

- Serve the burgers by topping them with the delicious lemon butter and green mash.

Note: Does not mix too thoroughly as it can make burgers tough. For additional flavors, you can add garlic, chili, or your favorite herbs.

Keto dinner recipes

Going easy on keto diet seems impossible to many, but this is not the case. You can have your favorite meals with little alterations in the ingredients. You can still enjoy your romantic dinners or dinners with family by following our keto-friendly dinner recipes.

1. *Keto meatballs*

Being on the keto diet and making yourself a meat dish which obeys the laws of the diet has not been complicated. Make this cheesy and delicious keto-friendly meatball dish for your dinner. Keto meal balls dish is a big YES on the keto diet.

Ingredients

For meatballs

- beef- 1lb (grounded)
- Egg- 1 (beaten)
- Garlic clove- 1 (minced)
- Mozzarella cheese ½ cup (shredded)
- Parmesan cheese- ¼ cup (grated)
- Kosher salt- to taste or 1 tsp
- Olive oil or butter- 2 tbsp

- Black pepper- to taste

For the sauce

- Garlic cloves- 2 (minced)

- Tomatoes- 1 (crushed)

- Onion- 1 (finely chopped)

- Dried oregano 1 tsp.

- Black pepper and sale- to taste

Directions

- Take a bowl and mix all the ingredients of the meatball. Form balls according to your desired size.

- Take a skillet and add olive oil, let the oil heat and then add the meatballs. Let them cook for 10 minutes. Take out the balls once done.

- In the same skillet add onion cook them until they become soft. Add minced garlic and cook for 1 minute. Add all other ingredients for the sauce and mix well.

- Add cooked meatballs into the sauce and let them simmer for 15 minutes.

- Before serving, garnish them with grated Parmesan cheese.

Note: Do not overcook the balls; they may become hard.

2. Keto Taco cups

Keto taco cups are the whole unique kind of keto dinner recipe which doubles your keto diet fun.

Ingredients

- Olive oil- 1 tbsp.

- Onion- 1 (chopped

- Garlic cloves- 3 (minced)

- Beef- 1lb (grounded)

- Cheddar cheese- 2 cups (grounded)

- Chili powder- 1 tbsp.

- Cumin- ½ tsp. (grounded)

- Paprika- ½ tsp.

- Salt and black pepper- to taste

For serving

- Cream

- Avocadoes

- Chopped cilantro

- Chopped tomatoes

Directions

- Preheat oven with a baking sheet and parchment paper.

- Add 2 tablespoons of cheddar cheese on the sheet and let the cheese melt. Wait until cheese becomes bubbly and its corners are getting golden.

- Take a muffin tin and spray cooking oil, and then pick the melted cheddar cheese and place at the bottom of the muffin tin. Fit with another inverted tin and wait until it gets chilly.

- If you do not have another tin, then you can use your hands to mold the cheese around the edges of the tin.

- Take a large skillet and add oil and onion. Cook until onion s get soft. Add garlic and cook for 1 minute. Add beef and cook for 6 minutes.

- Drain the fat and again put the meat into the same skillet and add chili powder, cumin, salt, pepper, and paprika.

- Transfer the ready cheese cups to serving the dish and fill them with cooked meat. Top with sour cream, chopped avocados, cilantro, and tomatoes.

3. Keto Bacon Sushi

Keto bacon sushis are the ultimate solution to your bacon cravings. They add a lot of ingredients, but they are in line with your keto diet requirements, i.e., high in fat and low on carbs!

Ingredients

- Bacon- 6 (halved)

- Carrots- 2 (thinly sliced)

- Avocado-1 (sliced)

- Cucumbers- 2 (sliced)

- Cream cheese- 4 oz.

- Sesame seeds

Directions

- Preheat oven at 400°. Spread baking sheet and aluminum foil into the cooking rack. Place halved bacon onto the sheet until they become crispy.

- Cut all the vegetables according to the size of bacon.

- When bacon gets cold, then add layers of cream cheese on each slice of bacon.

- Spread vegetables on the bacon. Roll up all the vegetables tightly.

- Garnish it with the sesame seeds and satisfy your appetite.

Keto smoothie recipes

Fruits are the favorites of many, and a lot of people do not want to give up on fruits during their keto diet- they don't even need to! Make keto-friendly smoothies for yourself and enjoy healthy living!

1. Keto Green smoothie

Keto green smoothie is what you need to keep yourself refreshing, healthy, and energetic. Make yourself this smoothie and have all the nutrients which you need during your keto diet.

Ingredients

- Spinach- a handful or according to need

- Coconut milk- 1 glass (unsweetened)

- Avocados- 1

- Vanilla extract- to taste

Directions

- Add all the ingredients into a blender and blend well until smooth.

- Pour into a glass and garnish it with keto-friendly nuts.

- You can add ice cubes to have chilled one.

2. *Keto cucumber lime smoothie*

Cucumber lime smoothie all what you need for your keto goals. It is not only delicious but nutritious! If you are looking for something refreshing, then this smoothie is for you. It keeps you hydrated on the keto diet.

Ingredients

- Celery- a bunch

- Cucumber- ½

- Lime- 1 tbsp

- Water- to need

- Ice

Directions

- Blend all the ingredients well and add ice for adding some extra taste.

- If you feel like, you can squeeze the lemon into it (if you like the extra lime taste).

- Drink and have a refreshing time.

3. Matcha Collagen Smoothie

Match Collagen a powerhouse smoothie which comes with all the essential nutrients which one requires during the keto diet. You can start your day with this great smoothie and stay refreshing all day.

Ingredients

- Almond milk

- Coconut milk

- Avocado

- Mint

- Cilantro

- Lime

- Vanilla

- Ice

Directions

- Blend all the ingredients well and serve smoothie chilled.

- Avocados are essential in the smoothie because they make the smoothie thicker and creamier.

4. Keto blueberry ginger smoothie

The blueberry ginger smoothie is considered as excellent for boosting up the ketone levels of a person. Hence it is a must-to-have smoothie on the keto diet. The smoothie is nutritious and full of taste. You can add it to your breakfast and enjoy the whole day with full energy.

Ingredients

- Blueberries

- Coconut milk

- Apple

- Collagen powder

- MCT oil

- Stevia

- Ginger

- Coconut yogurt

Directions

- Blend all the ingredients well and keep a check on the proportion of ingredients.

- Add an appropriate amount of all the ingredients to get optimum benefits.

Keto Snack Recipes

Being on a keto diet and satisfying your snacks craving is not a challenging one. You can make keto-friendly snacks to help you with your addictions. Make yourself these delicious and nutritious snacks and enjoy your keto journey!

1. Salad sandwiches

As bread is a big no in the keto diet, then you must be thinking about how we are going to make sandwiches without bread? If yes, then we have the alternative to make sandwiches with!

Ingredients

- Romaine lettuce- 2oz.
- Butter- ½ oz.
- Cheese- 1 oz.
- Cherry tomatoes- 1
- Avocado- ½

Directions

- Thoroughly wash the lettuce. Consider it as a base for your sandwiches.

- Smear butter over the lettuce. Spread cheese, tomatoes, and avocado over the top.

- You can add other toppings as well according to your desire. You can add egg white or cooked tuna.

2. *Keto tortilla pizza*

Who does not love pizza? But with keto, you may need to be careful to have a typical pizza. But there is nothing to worry about even on the keto diet you can have a keto-friendly pizza.

Ingredients

For tortilla

- Egg whites- 2

- Eggs- 2

- Cream cheese- 6 oz.

- Husk powder- 1 tsp. (grounded)

- Coconut flour- 1 tbsp.

For topping

- Cheese- 2 cups (shredded)

- Tomato sauce- ½ cup

- Dried oregano- 2 tsp.

- Salt and pepper- to taste

Directions

For tortillas

- Preheat the oven at 400°F (200°C).

- Whisk the egg whites and eggs well in a bowl for 2 minutes. Add cream cheese and mix well until you get a smooth batter.

- Take salt, husk powder, and coconut flour and mix them well. Start adding the mixed powder into the batter. Whisk well to make the smooth batter.

- Take two baking sheets and place parchment paper over each of them.

- Spread the batter evenly. Bake for 5 minutes or wait until the tortilla starts turning into brown color.

For pizza

- Turn oven on at 450°F (225°C).

- Take tortillas and start spreading tomato paste, sauce, salt and pepper on each tortilla. Spread the shredded cheese over the toppings. Bake the pizza until cheese melts thoroughly.

- Take out your tortilla pizza and enjoy.

3. *Caprese snack*

The Caprese snacks are full of pleasant aromas, making you droll. You can take it as a snack or even as an appetizer.

Ingredients

- Cherry tomatoes- 8 oz.

- Mozzarella cheese- 8 oz.

- Green pesto- 2 tbsp.

- Salt and pepper- to taste

Directions

- Cut mozzarella cheese and tomato balls half wise.

- Add pesto and stir thoroughly.

- Sprinkle salt and pepper over it.

- You can add basil or parsley leaves to add extra colors to your snacks.

Intermittent fasting

Chapter 1: Introduction to intermittent fasting

Intermittent fasting is more natural than most of the other dietary plans. With nominal efforts, you can enjoy the benefits of IF without counting calories, eliminating specific food items from your diet or meal preparations. You are merely required not to eat or eat in a limit for a particular time.

There are many ways you can do IF. Some IF experts are in favor of time-restricted ingestion, allowing eating only for eight to ten hours a day with an overnight fast of fourteen to sixteen hours. Others emphasize the benefits of the 5:2 diet. This diet lets you enjoy your regular meals five days a week, whereas you can have only 25% of your daily calories intake. This number of calories is around 500 to 600 calories on average. Another opinion is to skip eating altogether on several days of the week. Only water, tea, or black coffee can be taken to satisfy the hunger pangs.

Intermittent fasting is a routine of eating rather than a diet. It requires you to schedule your mealtimes in the way which lets you get the most out of them. It is not about what type of food you take; it is all about when you have it.

Intermittent fasting is a popular way to shed your extra pounds and enhance the overall health and vitality nowadays. It is a method to schedule fasting and eating appropriately.

Intermittent fasting is not a new thing, but there are evidence that it was practiced as a health secret in ancient times. This powerful health secret was long-lost until recently when people rediscovered it, and it started being popular once again.

The number of internet searches made for "intermittent fasting" has amplified by around 10,000 percent, especially in the previous few years. If practiced appropriately, intermittent fasting has enormous potential to reduce excess weight, improving digestion system, controlling type2 diabetes, and much more. It does not require you to spend money on fancy diet items, spend time to count calories, and is extremely simple to follow.

The purpose of this guide is to facilitate you about every aspect of intermittent fasting; you may need to know as a beginner.

Why Is Intermittent Fasting a better diet plan?

Intermittent fasting is a great way to get slim without being on a crash diet or lowering your calorie intake into nothing. When you start intermittent fasting, you attempt to keep your food the same as in your routine. Mostly, people tend to eat more for a shorter time. This way, intermittent fasting helps to maintain muscle mass while you lose weight.

Most people go for intermittent fasting to lose excessive fat. We will have a look at how intermittent fasting causes weight loss.

The foremost reason is that intermittent fasting is the most natural strategy. You can opt for losing your extra fat while maintaining the muscle mass is that it does not require drastic changes in your behavior. This quality makes it a more manageable diet plan, which could be followed for a prolonged time frame.

Intermittent fasting is not starvation because it is a deliberate effort to control your food intake for a certain period, unlike hunger, when the absence of food is not in your control. Starvation is a too long and involuntary break from eating, which may result in serious health issues and sometimes, even death. On the other hand, fasting is a way to put your body on breaks from eating only as long as they do not put you under any health risk. Moreover, food is available, but you do not eat it by choice rather than by force for a while suitable for your body's requirements. You may start your fast any time and for as long as you want. There is no standard duration for fasting. You can decide the most suitable length after consulting your physician.

You are already fasting when you are not eating. For example, the duration between your dinner and breakfast, which is most of the time, around 12 to 14 hours can also be called intermittent fasting. This makes intermittent fasting a routine affair. You have breakfast to break the fast you started after your dinner, and you do it daily. This fact has another implication also that you should make fasting a part of your routine, even if it is for a short period.

There is nothing unusual and strange about intermittent fasting, but it is a very reasonable part of your daily life. You may call it the most powerful and oldest diet plan through human history, but somehow, we could not benefit from its potential to the fullest.

The mechanism of Intermittent Fasting

To understand how we can lose weight with intermittent fasting, we must be clear about the difference between the fasted and fed state of the body.

While eating, digesting, and absorbing the nutrients, your body is in the fed state. Usually, this state begins when you eat and goes on for three to five hours until your body has digested and absorbed the meal you just had. Due to the higher level of insulin during the fed state, it is challenging for your body to burn fat.

After this duration, the body enters the post-absorptive state, which means, your body has already processed the meal. This state lasts till around eight to twelve hours after eating, which is when you begin the fasted state. With a lower level of insulin during this state, your body can burn the fat quickly in the fasted state.

Your body can burn the fat in a fasted state, which was inaccessible through the fed state.

Our bodies are rarely in this fat-burning state because it takes almost twelve hours after eating to enter the fasted state. This is the reason behind people losing fat during intermittent fasting even without any particular change in the amount and frequency of eating and exercise schedule. Fasting leads your body into the fat-burning state, which rarely occurs during our routine eating schedule. Understanding what happens to your body when you eat is crucial to know how intermittent fasting works. When we eat, a hormone called insulin releases into our body, but it is not required all the time. Your insulin level goes down to a typically average level while fasting, enabling you to consume your stored body fat. So, weight loss is impossible without getting the insulin level down. This is the reason why consuming frequent small meals does not let you lose weight.

Different Types of Intermittent Fasting Schedules

Here are a few points for you if you are planning to give intermittent fast a try to make it a part of your routine.

Leangains Model of intermittent fasting is considered the best model. It involves eight hours of eating and sixteen hours fast in a day. Martin Berkhan of Leangains.com popularize this model, and it is the origin for the name of this model. It is also called the 8/16 method of intermittent fasting. The critical rule is that you have to skip your breakfast daily.

When to start doesn't matter if you go for an eight hours diet time. You may begin at 1 pm till 11 pm or if you like, starting at 7 am and stopping at 3 pm is also a good option. Pick whatever suits you. In many cases, eating from1 pm to 8 pm goes well as these times let me enjoy my lunch and dinner with friends and family. I usually take my breakfast alone, so skipping it isn't a big deal for me.

Intermittent fasting becomes a habit quickly because you practice it daily. Currently, you may have an eating schedule without feeling it. Well, intermittent fasting is just the same with only requiring you not to eat at particular times, which are a walk in the park.

But because you usually skip one or two meals a day, maintaining the same calorie intake during the week may be a tedious task for most of the people. In simple words, it's challenging to have bigger meals consistently. As a result, a large number of people trying this style of intermittent fasting manage to lose weight eventually. If you intend to lose weight, this is an advantage of intermittent fasting, but otherwise, it's not your cup of tea.

Sharing my experience, I have been following intermittent fasting throughout the previous year, but I am not crazy about my diet. I focus on adopting healthy habits, which can lead my 90 % behavior, allowing me to do whatever I want in the remaining 10 %. I may enjoy my favorite fast food anytime and balance it next time with fasting because I enjoy the flexibility of my diet plan.

Weekly Intermittent Fasting

As a beginner, fasting once a week or once a month is an excellent way to start your intermittent fasting routine. Even this occasional fasting can give you the benefits you expect from regular fasting. Besides losing weight, there are many other health benefits you may get from starvation. If your lunch on Monday is your last meal and you fast until lunchtime on Tuesday, you are skipping only two meals a day. Because you are not cutting much on your calorie intake, you aren't going to lose any weight. This makes it a fantastic option if you want to maintain your weight.

There are many ways to incorporate twenty-four hours of fasting in your routine. You may like to have it after a hearty feast with friends and family or just after a long traveling adventure.

This twenty-four hours fasting is a great way to motivate you for intermittent fasting in the future. Once done successfully, you are brave enough to survive smaller fasting durations after twenty-four hours fast. It lifts the mental barrier of being hungry for so long, enabling you to try for more health adventures of this kind.

Alternate Day Intermittent Fasting

This type of intermittent fasting involves prolonged fasting sessions on alternate days throughout the week. The other name for this plan is the eat-stop-eat method.

For instance, you may have dinner on Friday night and then stop eating until Saturday evening. On Sunday, though, you may eat as and how you like the entire day. Your fast will start again after dinner on Sunday. This method has more consistency because you have a minimum of one meal a day. Once getting habitual, this method is straightforward to follow because of its flexibility.

But even then, this style of intermittent fasting is more famous for research purposes than in real life. The reason may be the longer duration of fasting, which may not be easy to follow for everyone. Moreover, eating only for dinners deprives you of all the fun you may want to have while dining out for lunches within your social circle.

This style is the best if you are looking for a diet plan to shed your extra calories because you have longer hours of fasted state than in the Leangains method of fasting.

Based on research, adopting the habit of eating bigger meals in routine is the toughest part of the alternated day fasting style. You can enjoy a delicious meal once a while is alright. But teaching your body to have the same heavy meal requires planning, loads of ready to eat food and to eat steadily. The final result is that people who try intermittent fasting end up shedding some extra fat. This happens because the quantity of their meals remains the same despite cutting out a few meals weekly.

Warrior diet was introduced by Ori Hofmekler. This fasting style allows eating only four hours of feeding time. You have to consume your entire routine food in only four hours while fasting for the remaining twenty hours.

Taking the amount of food you usually consume within twenty-four hours in just four hours may cause indigestion or uncomfortable stomach conditions because of over-eating. This is an extreme method of fasting, and you must proceed to it after having built stamina to survive longer fasting hours. Since it allows very less eating time, the calorie intake automatically reduces, which results in weight loss. Maintaining your current or losing your excess weight isn't a problem when you are on intermittent fasting. Managing weight in any way is not at all an issue while following the fasting diet schedule. However, if you choose to fast for twenty-four hours on multiple days per week, you may find it challenging to eat enough on your cheat days to make up for the calorie count you lose while fasting.

So, you may choose from intermittent daily fasting, twenty-four hours once a week or once per month according to the suitability and requirements of your body. A large number of people opt for the 16/8 method because it is the most sustainable, most straightforward, and most comfortable to follow.

Since you eat in a controlled way by limiting eating time, you must lose weight as a result of intermittent fasting, whatever method you choose to schedule it. The weight loss is mandatory in intermittent fasting because you can rarely have the same calorie intake you eat otherwise when you are not fasting.

Whatever method you pick, the rule is, either you cannot eat anything or have some tea, coffee, or water to kill the hunger and keep yourself dehydrated.

Where to begin?

After having discussed what intermittent fasting is and how it works, now is the time to see how to get started.

Whichever method you pick for intermittent fasting, keep one thing in mind, it is always challenging to get used to your controlled eating schedule.

You may experience low energy level, low blood pressure, mood swings anxiety, or even headache in some cases because your body is not accustomed to skipping meals.

Most of the fasters go through uncomfortable feeling of hollowness, low blood sugar level, or lightheadedness due to lack of food intake. Others may have dizziness and lack of focus and concentration.

 Moreover, you may try various methods of intermittent fasting before selecting the one which works best for you. Consider your goals in terms of weight loss or maintaining weight, work routine, and other health effects of fasting on your body.

The best way, to begin with, is to limit your eating time from free period to first twelve hours. You may proceed to reduce it further once your body gets used to it. Stop where you find it most appropriate to follow consistently. People who have physical work or work outdoors for long hours may consider a fasting method which does not require them to skip meals during the day. This schedule must also allow the liquid intake to stay hydrated through the working hours.

Usually, it takes your body a month to get adapted to the new routine of controlled eating time. Your body adjusts itself according to your method, unlike the restricted calorie diet where you keep eating in small portions after shorter intervals. You may begin with an overnight fast, which is easier to manage because you don't need a high energy level to perform your routine duties as you spend most of the night sleeping. Research has proved that overnight fasting adjusts eating patterns with a daily schedule of eating and helps to promote weight loss and better metabolism.

Tips for intermittent fasting

You don't have to watch your calorie count while being on intermittent fast but only restrict the period when you can cherish your delicious meals. It's more about time rather than the number of calories you consume. You don't need to follow any hard and fast rules on what type of food you can eat or which food group to avoid.

Set a goal:

There is always a purpose of starting intermittent fasting, which may be weight loss, improved metabolism or improve overall health. Select a target and estimate your daily calorie intake accordingly.

Consult your physician

Consult your doctor before starting intermittent fasting, particularly if you have blood pressure issues, diabetes, or any other chronic health condition.

Consider your body and its needs

Always start with shorter periods of fasting and let your body adjust to the change.

Keep your work routine in your mind and arrange calorie intake and rehydration methods accordingly.

Stop fasting if you suffer from extreme dizziness, lack of concentration, or any other physical issue.

Choose the most suitable method

Try various methods of intermittent fasting to see which ones your body gets along in the most appropriate.

Estimate calories need

If you are fasting to lose weight, estimate the number of calories you need to perform your daily tasks effectively. On the other hand, if you are already underweight, plan your diet in a way that you could consume sufficient healthy calories within your eating time. You may use some digital method to maintain your calorie record. You may consult your dietician to have a better idea of how many calories you need to maintain a healthy lifestyle.

Plan your meals

Although there are no restrictions on amount or type of food and you can consume during intermittent fasting, yet you should plan your meals, including a healthy diet full of fiber and nutrients. This meal plan helps you follow your calorie count.

Choose healthy food options

Your body has already a shorter time period to consume the necessary nutrients so; it is a great step to consider the nutritional value of the food you consume. Avoid empty calories and opt for fresh food. Processed food is not a good option because it contains chemicals and preservatives.

Disadvantages and Side Effects of Intermittent fasting

Suffering from hunger is a significant issue in intermittent fasting. Desire further causes low blood pressure, sugar, and insulin level, which may lead to weakness and dizziness. But don't worry, your body will soon get used to it.

Women who are trying to conceive, have a history of amenorrhea, are pregnant, or breastfeeding must not go for longer fasted states because it may cause serious health issues for them. But if you are a healthy adult, you may go for intermittent fasting anytime you want.

Chapter 2:

Chapter 2 importance of intermittent fasting

Intermittent fasting can boost health in many ways if done appropriately. There are facts proven by various research studies that it affects human well-being positively.

Effects on Hormones and Cells

Fasting affects the cellular and molecular processes of your body. Your body produces hormones to burn the stored fat for producing energy when you are not eating for more extended periods.

The human growth hormone or HGH increases during intermittent fasting up to five times. This increase in HGH promotes muscle gain and fat loss.

As mentioned earlier, insulin levels decrease during the fasted state. Consequently, the stored fat in the body is consumed to run the system.

Our body produces free radicals, which damage the vital body cells like DNA and protein. This process leads to aging and many chronic diseases. Intermittent fasting enhances the resistance against oxidative stress according to many health studies. Mostly, oxidative stress occurs when there are many toxins accumulated in your body. Intermittent fasting detoxes your body by burning excessive fat and bad cells.

The cells also start repairing the damages and modify the genes expression. This repairing process is called autophagy. During autophagy, cells eliminate the wastage, including dysfunctional and old proteins gathered inside the cells. The genes expressions are modified about immunity and longevity. These variations lead to better internal processes and the reduced aging process.

Intermittent fasting turbocharges your cells in many ways. It improves the regenerative capabilities of the stem cells. On the other hand, it reduces the destruction of mitochondria too. Mitochondria are called the powerhouse of your body cells. If they are healthy, your body will be automatically healthy.

Simplifying the routine

You don't have to worry about your breakfast and in some cases about lunch as well when fasting. Moreover, you don't have to count calories if you want to lose weight because you have restricted time for eating. So, no more stress of what to eat makes life simple along with saving your cooking time.

Increasing lifespan

Controlling calorie intake is a proven way to prolong the lifespan. Intermittent fasting triggers several processes which slow down the wear and tear in your body. As a result, the aging process slows down.

Reducing the Risk of Cancer

Intermittent fasting detoxifies the body by burning the extra and damaged cells. Cancer is a disease of unwanted growth of cells in the body. Controlled eating during the intermittent fasting decreases the growth of these harmful cells in your body. The two ways process of detoxification and restricted growth of cells has the potential to reduce the risk of cancer to some extent.

The easiest diet plan

Most people cannot follow a diet plan for a long time. This happens because almost every diet allows only a few food types which become boring a few days after starting. For example, in the ketogenic diet, you cannot eat carbohydrates or fats. This means, no bread, pasta, pizza, and sweets.

Moreover, our body needs all the food groups to work correctly. Intermittent fasting allows you to eat whatever you want but within the restricted time. This is an inclusive diet schedule, and you can prepare your meals according to your taste.

Lower stress level

In a typical dieting and intermittent fasting is that planning meals, keeping a strict check on calorie intake, the elimination of your favorite foods from the diet, hunger pangs and the feeling of deprivation causes stress and depression. This depression again results in excessive eating, which ruins all the effort done to control the weight. You can enjoy your favorite sweet dish, snack, or comfort food with carbohydrates any time before you start the fast again.

The flexibility which intermittent fasting allows as compared to the other restricted diet plans gives you a sense of freedom and autonomy. The only thing you take care of is the duration of your eating. The motivation level of the people practicing intermittent fasting is found high during a study in comparison to those following other diet plans.

Weight loss

Dieting for weight loss has become a cliché nowadays. Most people start dieting because they want to lose weight. You consume fewer meals, which automatically reduces the calorie intake. Moreover, you have to quit eating after a certain period until you break your fast. This practice again restricts the amount of food you eat. Consequently, your body has to burn the already stored fat, which results in weight loss.

Along with that, as mentioned above, intermittent fasting activates the hormones promoting weight loss. Additionally, decreasing insulin level in the blood, it intensifies the release norepinephrine, which is a fat-burning hormone. This hormone may increase the metabolic rate from three to fourteen times.

A study conducted in 2014 found that intermittent fasting can root three to eight percent weight loss within a time of three to twenty weeks. This change is noteworthy as compared to the other diet plans. The same study concluded that people who lost weight through intermittent fasting reduced their waist circumference as well. This reduction in their waist measurement means they lost their belly fat also, which is considered the most stubborn fat to cut. This fat doesn't only look bad but also causes diseases of the vital organs. This way, intermittent fasting can reduce the risk of potential heart, lungs, and stomach and kidney diseases.

Weight loss is not only about looking beautiful and fit, but it protects you from many diseases as well. Heart issues, joint pains, and diabetes are some diseases which you can get if you are overweight. Intermittent fasting helps you to reduce the risk of such diseases by healthily reducing weight.

You lose lesser muscle mass during intermittent fasting than any other way of calorie-restricted diet according to another research.

All these factors boost the weight loss process and make intermittent fasting one of the best weight-loss strategies. But if you manage to eat full of calories, more substantial meals even during intermittent fasting, you may gain weight instead of losing any of your accumulated body fat.

Reduced risk of type2 diabetes

Due to the lower release of insulin in the blood, there are fewer chances of type 2 diabetes when you are fasting. Intermittent fasting can lower blood sugar level by up to six percent and insulin level by thirty percent. These facts and figures must lead to protection and control of type 2 diabetes. So, if you have a history of diabetes in your family or diagnosed as a pre-diabetes patient, intermittent fasting can help you stay healthy.

The weight you lose as a result of intermittent fasting makes you insulin sensitive and keeps the blood sugar level down.

Inflammation

Your body loses damaged cells and waste during intermittent fasting, and this way reduces inflammation. Inflammation is mostly caused by the toxic materials gathered in the human body, and it may lead to severe and chronic health issues. Inflammation of soft tissues include liver, intestines, kidneys, and lungs inflammation, which may be fatal. By removing toxins from your body and reducing inflammation, intermittent fasting helps you stay safe from the potential risk of such ailments.

Improved heart health

Increased level of LDL or bad cholesterol, blood triglycerides, and inflammation are the risk factors for heart disease. Excessive body weight is also interlinked with heart problems, which can be effectively controlled by intermittent fasting.

Increased Brain health

The brain hormone BDNF increases as a result of intermittent fasting. This hormone is responsible for the growth of nerve cells. This way, all the brain diseases which are caused by the slow growth of new brain cells can be overcome. Alzheimer's disease is a chronic brain problem which gradually leads towards the memory loss and loss of coordination in the movement of various body parts. The scientists still have not discovered any effective treatment for it. The only way to stay safe is to protect against it. This new growth of brain cells boosted by intermittent fasting can prevent you from Alzheimer's disease.

As intermittent fasting reduces inflammation of the soft tissues, it affects the brain as well. So, the local conditions of swelling of the brain and the problems caused by them can be controlled to some extent through intermittent fasting.

Parkinson's disease is also a dangerous brain condition which develops slowly and cannot be cured. Just like Alzheimer's disease, the only way to protect against it is to promote the growth of new brain cells. Intermittent fast protects you from Parkinson's disease by helping in the growth of healthy nerve cells.

Intermittent fasting helps you to improve memory as well according to other research.

Managing body clock

Intermittent fasting affects the body clock or circadian rhythm also. You have set time for eating and fast, which helps your body schedule your sleep and wake timing. Moreover, consuming food long before going to bed prevents you from acid refluxes. It takes a while before your body adjusts itself according to your eating schedule. But once done, it brings positive changes in your sleep quality, timing, and activity level.

Faster metabolism

Intermittent fasting triggers your metabolism wonderfully. As a result of the improved metabolic effectiveness, the glycogen level in your body is discarded. This, in turn, activates the burning of fatty acids. This active metabolism due to intermittent fasting is a symbol of a healthy and energetic body.

Better immunity system

The immunity system of our bodyguards us against the diseases we may catch anytime from our surroundings. It works better if our body is not loaded with unwanted toxins. Intermittent fasting removes the toxins and the waste produced by the metabolism of our body. This way, it helps us maintain a stronger immune system to fight against potential diseases.

In addition to the above-mentioned benefits, there are many positive impacts of intermittent fasting, which you can discover for yourself. Fasting gives you positivity, focus, and peace of mind. Your life gets systemized while you are fasting because you have to organize your eating, work, and sleep routine. The habits developed this way can become a part of your personality and may help you excel in our professional life as well.

Chapter 3: Problems of obesity among women and how intermittent fasting solve these problems

Obesity is in the top 10 list of problematic factors of the whole world. No one wants to be obese. (Obesity is the slight overweight or the fat in random places that can make your beautiful body look ugly.) This trait is most commonly found in women because of their short heights and extreme diets. However, women are 99% of the population that are worried about being obese.

Obesity is also the primary (source) reason that women get prone to many diseases. Just like women are weak in front of sweets and sweet, adorable things, women get a considerable risk of diabetes due to obesity. It will lead to a major issue as to causing heart diseases or cancers.

In this modern era of the hustle and bustle, and sitting on the computer for several hours each day, exercise is a godsend. We humans are not designed to sit on our butts for so many hours each day. Our bodies eventually become weaker and become immune to diseases.

One of the most common diseases in the world is obesity. Some people don't even consider obesity as an issue. Of course, you should learn to love your body. It's a blessing. You're one out a million others that even got a body, to begin with. The other 999,999 didn't also get a body. If that isn't a blessing, I wonder what is.

But yeah, if you're obese and want to change your body type, you're on the right track.

Dangers of Obesity

Obesity is linked to a lot of dangerous diseases/health issues. Here are some of them:

Type-2 Diabetes - Diabetes isn't a disease. It's a condition. Diabetes is a condition where the blood sugar level is too high. It can cause significant heart diseases, kidney diseases, and maybe even lead to stroke, amputation, or blindness. Diabetes kills a lot of people these days.

Heart Diseases - Having excessive fat in your body can cause some of your nerves to get stressed or even damage the area around your heart. This can lead to you developing a lot of diseases.

Stroke – Having excessive fat can cause your body to be more prone to strokes. Strokes are not to be dealt with lightly. They're highly dangerous.

Cancer – Obesity has been linked to increasing the risk of developing cancer. Fat cells may release hormones that affect cell growth that'll eventually lead to cancer. Some of these cancers include breast cancer, colon/rectum cancer, kidney cancer, gallbladder cancer, and even uterus cancer.

Osteoarthritis – Osteoarthritis is a health issue that is linked to severe pain in the joints. Sometimes the joints get so stiff that it can become physically dangerous for a person to move them around frequently.

Pregnancy Problems – Your health can affect your child's health too. If you're a female, pregnant, and obese, it will have a terrible effect on the child's health.

Aside from all the dangers, you will be safe from, by slimming down, you'll also be able to look and feel better. You'll live longer, have a better friends circle, and the whole world's attention will be at your knees. You'll become a better person overall, too, and the risks of developing psychological diseases like depression or anxiety will decrease by a lot. If you're still looking to stay fat, that's totally up to you, but there are almost no benefits to staying obese, except that you'll become a good meat shield in case of a battle. If you're looking to slimmer down, the first thing you can try is doing cardio.

Cardio – the obesity killer

Cardio is short for cardiovascular exercise. In a very general sense of the definition, cardio means literally anything that makes your heart race and makes you breathe hard. NO, looking at your crush isn't cardio. If it were, I would be as toned as Jeff from Athlean-X. Anyways, in a better sense of the word, doing any kind of exercise that raises your blood pressure and heart rate is cardio.

 The most basic of all exercises for cardio is running. Everyone can run. We've all run at one point in our lives.

Running for Cardio

Yes, running for cardio may seem like an effort. To see sound effects, you will need to cardio for a long duration. Though it may be inefficient, you can run at your own pace. You don't need to use 100% of your strength all the time while running. Even jogging is a good alternative to running, for cardio.

Who should run: people who don't suffer from Osteoarthritis should run. Running is also a very good exercise that allows you to build stamina and reduce sweat when running away from danger. Running away is a very tactical move. Everyone should know how to be efficient at running.

Weight training for Cardio

Lifting weights is an excellent way to lose calories and gain right muscle on your body. Not only are you losing weight, but you're also gaining good muscle. In other words, you're doing two good things at the same time. When you've lost all your weight, you'll look better than your peers who lost their weight through running or any simple interval training.

Who should lift weight: People who have no issue dedicating an hour at the gym every day should lift the weight. If you have problems breathing, or issues dealing with intensity exercises, you should refrain from hitting the gym until your doctor agrees to do so. Weight lifting has been linked with an increase in confidence and other good psychological effects too, by the way.

Doing yoga

Okay, hear me out. Some people are really skeptical of yoga even being an exercise, but many people have seen positive results by doing yoga on a regular basis. Firstly introduced in India, and then spread to the rest of the result of the world, yoga is an art.

Heck, a review of 17 studies done by Larson Meyer has revealed that doing yoga is as useful as doing a high-intensity workout. Yes, you won't hear loud screaming or teeth grinding in your yoga classes, but you'll definitely see people losing weight and getting better at moving their body around.

 Don't try doing yoga at home for the first time, though. Join a Yoga class and thoroughly learn how to do Yoga. The poses are everything.

Who should do yoga: Everyone should do yoga. Yoga is even recommended at some hospital centers where patients have joint issues. Yoga is a mystical art that helps release the pain and tension, in-between the joints and helps your body stretch and move more. If you have physical problems, you can stay away from certain yoga poses. But overall, I think everyone can do yoga.

Intermittent Fasting

If you do not wish to employ cardio training to lose extra fat, things like intermittent fasting will definitely help you perform better, for cheaper. Fasting comes at a low risk too, so you can expect a lot of performance and other boosts while you're on your fasting time period.

Advantages of fasting

Here is a list of benefits for fasting:

Cheap

Fasting is really cheap and doesn't really cause a big hole in your wallet. In fact, fasting helps you protect against a lot of financial issues too, such as buying food for breakfast, lunch, brunch and dinner and other snacks.

There are different types of fasts, but the most common one is the Muslim fast that involves your fasting from the first ray of sunshine in the morning to the fall of the sun in the evening. It should last from 12 to 18 hours, depending on where you live.

Religious

Fasting is considered a part of religion among several religious associations. This is because fasting has a really good effect on one's body. Religion is all about love and doing stuff that is super good for one's personal and social life. Religion, at its core, is preaching love.

Anyone can do it

Unlike cardio or yoga, which involves physical labor, fasting can be done by anyone. Whether you're a person with no legs or just an overly obese person who can't even walk without having extreme pain in your joints, fasting is for everyone. Everyone can do it, and no one should have any issues with it.

Don't hurt yourself

The most important thing when working out or planning your diet is the fact that you might end up hurting yourself in the process. Do not do that. You can follow a specific regime given to you by a trusted physician or diet planner that will help you diet better and safer.

Keep your diet balanced

If you want to keep yourself healthy, and working, keep your diet balanced. Do not always eat Magnesium or Protein. Eat carbs and natural fats too. Don't stop eating sugar. Your body still needs sugar for quick energy. And your taste buds too. After all, what's a life without a little spice and a little sugar, right?

Keto Diet with Fasting

You can keep a keto diet while fasting too. A keto diet is a fantastic diet that involves a high fat, low carb diet, and you'll start seeing results before long.

By not eating the whole day, and then doing Keto Diet, you'll be losing weight faster than Adele's balls rolling on the ground. And yes, that's fast. Very fast, indeed.

You'll be helping the world

By doing fasting, you're doing a better job at helping the world become a better place. Not consuming resources means that fewer resources of the world have to be harvested to quench your hunger. If everyone did a fast every now and then, our world's food resources usage would be cut by quite a lot and making it easier to solve world hunger. Sure, that may seem like a long haul, but it does work. Trust me. I did the maths. I like maths after all.

Consult your physician

Before beginning this diet, do consult your physician and your diet planner to check if the diet works out perfectly for you. The physician knows better than we do about your body. Some of the factors of fasting may not be suited for everyone, and they can give you physical scars. Work on protecting yourself from that.

Better performance

It has been scientifically proved that fasting helps you perform better in the gym and overall when working in the office or in the school.

Though the first few days might seem like hell, once your body gets used to it, it'll become more efficient at doing its tasks.

Some extra benefits:

Here are some of the things that change in your body when you fast:

Insulin: Insulin increases when we eat food. When we fast, the levels of insulin in our body decreases dramatically. Lesser levels of insulin in our body dramatically facilitates fat burning.

Human growth hormone: Levels of growth hormone may go super high during a fast, up to as much as five times the average amount. Growth hormone is a hormone that can facilitate fat loss and help gain good muscle, among many other things.

Norepinephrine: The body's nervous system sends norepinephrine to the fat cells, making them break down body fat into fatty acids that can then be burned for energy. This is really useful for obese people.

How to start Intermittent Diet

Here are a few tips on starting the intermittent diet:

Some people fast on alternate days to improve weight loss gains. A person on the 5:2 method eats 500 to 600 calories on two not so consecutive days in each week of the day.

Some people even add in a third day of fasting each week. For the rest of the week, that person eats only the number of calories that they are burning during the day. Over time, this creates a calorie deficit that allows the person to lose weight as much as they want.

Figure out your calories

There are no dietary restrictions when fasting, but this does not mean that counting calories do not count. People who are wanting to lose weight need to specifically create a calorie deficit diet plan for themselves — this means that they need to know that they need to consume less energy than they use. People who are wanting to want to gain weight need to consume more calories than they already use. There are so many amazing tools available in the world that would help a person work out their caloric needs and determine how many calories they need to consume each day to either gain or lose weight. One can also converse with their healthcare provider or dietitian for guidance on how many calories they need.

A person interested in losing or gaining weight will find it easier to plan what they are going to eat during the day or week. Meal planning does not need to be overbearing. You just need to consider your calorie intake and then incorporating proper nutrients into that diet. Meal planning indeed does offer many benefits, such as helping a person stick to their calorie count, and ensuring they have the necessary food on hand for cooking recipes, quick meals, and snacks.

For a healthy, well-nourished person, intermittent fasting offers very few side effects. When a person first starts fasting, they may feel slightly physically and mentally sluggish as their body adjusts. After the adjustment, most people go back to functioning normally. However, people with medical conditions should consult their doctor before beginning any fasting program. People particularly at risk from fasting and who may require medical supervision include:

- women who are breastfeeding their children
- women who are pregnant with babies
- people who are trying to conceive a child
- people with the diabetes condition(type-2 or type-1)

- people who have difficulty regulating sugar (basically diabetes)

- people with low blood pressure (or even too high bp)

- people on medications related to eating disorders

- people who are underweight or malnourished

- people who are suffering from anorexia

Fasting is a very natural part of the human life cycle. People have done it since the beginning of time.

Many people have fasted throughout their lifetimes unknowingly: just by eating dinner early at night but skipping breakfast or vice versa. Many structured approaches may work well for some people, and you'll have to figure out what your body wants on your own. Do note that it is important to keep in mind that although a person does not need to exclude any specific food from their diet, they should still aim to eat a balanced diet which we discussed earlier. Remember to drink lots of water and soda once every month too. Finally, though any average Joe is a very likely experience no or minimal side effects, people with certain medical conditions or who are taking certain medications should learn to talk to their doctors before beginning this process.

Chapter 4: Intermittent diet recipes

Intermittent fasting breakfast recipes

A healthy and wishful breakfast is crucial in making the full day pass by happily and tension-free. Many people may crave to have substantial breakfast, but their diet plan does not allow them to do so. But even if you are on an intermittent fasting diet, you can still have wishful breakfast. Below are the breakfast recipes for people pursuing an intermittent fasting diet. All of the methods are the best one to satisfy the appetites of people following intermittent fasting diet.

Intermittent fasting diet followers can have their favorite meals while staying under boundaries.

1. *Intermittent fasting Caprese Omelet*

The Caprese Omelet can be made quickly and easily. The omelet is deliciously finger licking which fully satisfies the person having it. To make an omelet, you only require 10 minutes.

Ingredients

- Eggs- 3
- Oil- 1 tbsp
- Tomatoes- 1/3 cup
- Basil leaves- 5 (chopped)
- Parmesan cheese- ½ cup (grated)
- Pesto- 2tsps
- Salt and pepper- to taste

Directions

- Take out eggs in a bowl and whisk well.
- If necessary, add 1 tbsp of water.

- Heat the oil in a pan. Heat it.

- Pour the eggs and cook well. Tilt the pan a little so that uncooked egg can reach the edges.

- Once cooked, layer few tomatoes, parmesan cheese, and basil leave on the fried egg.

- Fold the egg and place it on the plate. Top the omelet with remaining tomatoes and pesto. Enjoy.

2. *Spinach and Feta Omelet*

Key to a perfect omelet is that it must not be overcooked. Make yourself a unique type of omelet. In the omelet, you can add your favorite toppings to make the perfect omelet for you within a few minutes. As for the topping, you can use cheese, olives, mushrooms, and tomatoes. One thing to note over here is that you can use one or two eggs instead of three if you don't feel starving. The preparation time which omelet takes is maximum of 15 minutes.

Ingredients

- Eggs- 2 or 3

- White mushrooms- 1 cup

- Feta cheese- 1/3 cup

- Garlic- 1 clove

- Olive oil- 2 tbsp

- Spinach- 3 cups

- Salt and pepper- to taste

Directions

- The first step is the preparation of filling. Take a pan and add olive oil in it, place garlic over it. Sprinkle salt and let the garlic cook for a minute. Then add white mushrooms and cook them for five minutes. Cook until mushrooms become brown.

- Now add spinach and cook for one to two minutes. Take out the mixture into the bowl. Clean the pan.

- Take a bowl and crack eggs in it. Stir thoroughly. Add salt and pepper in it.

- Heat the oil in the pan and pour whisked eggs mixture in it. Let the eggs cook. Tilt the pan to spread the uncooked egg to the corners.

- Don't overcook it so that it may end up crispy or dry. Make sure that egg remains soft.

- Once cooked, add already cooked mushroom mixture over it. Add crumbled feta.

- Fold the omelet and cook for another one minute. Dish out the delicious omelet and enjoy.

3. *Intermittent egg stuffed avocado*

Avocados are delicious yet healthy to pursue during the intermittent fasting diet. Egg yolks are enriched in vitamin A, B and D, minerals, and selenium. Eggs are not responsible for enhancing the blood cholesterol level. The time required for the preparation of the recipe is 5 minutes.

Ingredients

- Avocados- 2 (medium-sized)

- Eggs- 4

- Mayonnaise- ¼ cup

- Dijon Mustard- 1 tsp

- Salt- to taste

- Spring onions- 2

- Black pepper- to taste (grounded)

Directions

- First of all, boil the eggs. Take a saucepan and add water in it. Add a pinch of salt in it. Bring the water to boil. Now start dipping eggs into the boiling water. Wait for 10 minutes. After 10 minutes, turn off the flame. Place the eggs into the saucepan filled with cold water.

- Dice the eggs. Finely chop the spring onion.

- Take a bowl and mix the boiled eggs, sour cream, Dijon mustard, and mayonnaise. Garnish them with spring onions.

- Add salt and pepper and mix it well.

- Take avocados, cut them from half. Scoop the middle of avocados. Cut the scoop of avocados into beautiful pieces.

- Mix the finely chopped avocado pieces into the mixture.

- Take avocados and fill each avocado with egg mixture. Garnish with the spring onions and serve.

Intermittent fasting lunch recipes

People on the intermittent fasting diet have to be very specific in having their lunch. There are various choices under which a person can go for intermittent diet-friendly lunch. The diet is not about eating an only particular set of foods, but a person can add on a variety of ingredients and can enjoy his favorites with a blend of a few other ingredients. Here are the few intermittent fasting lunch recipes which you can make yourself.

1. *Avocado and bacon salad*

Avocados are very nutritious and are very good while being on a diet. They are known for boosting the electrolyte intake of the person. Moreover, they are high in fiber; that is why they are said to be best in the diet. This recipe takes overall 20 minutes for its preparation.

Ingredients

- Avocados- 2 (large)
- Lettuce- 2 (small)
- Fresh spinach- 2 cups
- Spring onion- 1 (medium size)
- Bacon- 4 large slices
- Eggs- 2 (optional)

Vinaigrette

- Virgin olive oil- 3 tbsp

- Apple cider vinegar- 1 tbsp

- Dijon mustard- 1 tsp

- Salt- to taste or a pinch

- Black pepper- to taste (freshly ground)

- Dash Tabasco (optional)

Note: try to get ingredients in their natural form. Try to avoid unnecessary additives in the ingredients.

Directions

- Take the bacon and a pan. Place the container over the stove and let it heat. Add oil and then place slices of bacon for crisping up. Once crisped up, add ½ cup of water in it and cook on medium flame. Medium heat is required to render the fat.

- Tear the lettuce and wash them well. Wash the spinach well. With the help of kitchen towel pat dry the spinach and lettuce. Halve the avocados and deseed them. Slice the avocados into stripes. Finely slice down all the avocados.

- For the vinaigrette, mix all the ingredients well. Take a bowl and add the virgin oil, apple cider vinegar, salt, pepper, Tabasco and Dijon mustard in it. Mix all of them well with the help of a spoon.

- (Optional step)- Take out a small saucepan and fill it to three quarters with water. Add a pinch of salt in it. Bring the water to boil. Once the water starts boiling, with the help of spoon or hand start adding eggs in it. Be careful while using hands. Let eggs cook for 10 minutes to boil them hard. Once eggs are boiled hard, remove them and put in the bowl filled with cold water. Peel off the eggs and slices them into small pieces.

- The next step is to assemble the salad. Take a salad bowl and start collecting by folding the spinach and lettuce. Torn the crisped bacon and add them into the salad bowl as well. Add sliced avocados and enjoy the delicious lunch.

2. Intermittent Italian Gnocchi soup

Many people in winters want to have soup as it is warm and nutritious. It helps in getting rid of various veggie clutters in your refrigerator. It is a traditional Italian soup, also known as Zuppa

Toscana. The preparation time which soup requires is almost 30 minutes. The recipe is to serve 4-6 persons.

Ingredients

- Italian sausage- 1 pound (ground)

- Small onion- 1 (small)

- Garlic- 2 cloves (minced)

- Chicken or beef bone broth- 4 cups

- Red pepper-1 (medium)

- Kale- 1 cup (chopped)

- Garlic gnocchi- 1 batch

- Heavy cream- ½ cup

- Salt- to taste

- Black pepper- to taste (ground)

- Parmesan cheese- (optional)

- Parsley- (optional)

- Crumbled bacon- (optional)

Directions

- Take a large stockpot or oven and heat it over medium-high heat. Add a little oil and heat it. Start adding onion, garlic and then sausages. Cook until the sausages become brown. Stir the sausages and break them with the help of a spoon. Once browned, drain out the excess of grease.

- Now add bone broth of beef or chicken and cook it for a minute. Then add diced red peppers into it. Let the mixture simmer well. Reduce the heat to low.

- Then add kale and cook it. Cook for another five minutes.

- Now add gnocchi and cream and mix it well.

- (Optional step) if you want to garnish it, then use parmesan cheese, parsley and crumbled bacon.

- Serve soup warm.

3. *Paleo pad thai recipe*

Another delicious yet on diet ingredient containing recipe is paleo pad thai one. The method is your diet-friendly and takes 30 minutes for the preparation. The recipe is favorite of many.

Ingredients

For sauce

- Fish sauce- ¼ cup

- Coconut aminos- 1 tbsp

- Sriracha- 1 tbsp (you can make your own)

- Garlic- 2 cloves

- Almond and cashew butter- 4 tbsp

- Salt- to taste

- Pepper- to taste (ground)

- Erythritol- 1 tbsp (optional)

- Liquid stevia- 5-7 drops (optional)

For stir-fry

- Chicken thighs- 500 g (boneless and skinless)

- Shirataki noodles- 2 packs

- Eggs- 4 large

- Spring onions- 2 medium

- Bean sprout- 2 cups

- Cilantro- ¼ cup (chopped)

- Flaked almonds- ¼ cup (toasted)

- Fresh lime juice- 2 tbsp

- Ghee pr virgin coconut oil- 1tbsp (oil) or ¼ cup ghee

- Shredded Red cabbage- 2 cups (optional)

Directions

- First of all, prepare the shirataki noodles. Wash the noodles and boil them to remove the natural odor. Once noodles are boiled, keep them in a bowl and set aside.

- Take a bowl and combine fish sauce, sriracha, coconut amino, crushed garlic, cashew butter, almond and salt, and pepper. Mix them well.

- Add erythritol or stevia in a bowl and set it aside.

- Cut the chicken thighs into one-inch pieces.

- Take a pan and add ghee or oil in it. Add chicken in it and cook over medium-high heat. Cook thoroughly. Mix the chicken well and cook until it becomes a little brown.

- You are once done set aside.

- Now prepare the omelet. Take a pan and add ½ tablespoon of ghee in it. Then add stirred eggs in it and let them cook.

- Make sure to whisk eggs well and then cook them well. Fill with the help of a spatula and cook for another 30 seconds. Once done, transfer it to the plate.

- Repeat the procedure for the next two eggs as well.

- Now roll up the omelet and cut it into strips. Slice the spring onion round and place them in a bowl which is filled with water. Clean the onion thoroughly. Now transfer on the kitchen towel and pat dry.

- Now place the chicken for cooking again and add spring onions. Cook over medium-high flame for two minutes. After two minutes, add omelet strips and cook for another one minute.

- Now add prepared sauce and noodles into the mixture. Mix thoroughly and turn off the heat.

- Once mixed well, add fresh cilantro.

- For serving, squeeze lime juice and toasted almonds.

- Garnish with red cabbage, cilantro, and lime wedges.

Note: to toast almond flakes, cook almond chips on the hot pan for one to two minutes over medium-high heat.

Intermittent fasting dinner recipes

Making an intermittent fasting diet-friendly dinner has never been as easy as it is with our guide. These recipes are the best one to follow to keep you within limits of the diet.

1. Intermittent chorizo meatballs

If you want to add extra taste to your lunchtime, then go for adding chorizos into your recipe. These chorizos will help you get rid of some of your excess pounds. If any of you is not a cheese enthusiast, then you can skip it. As meatballs are already moist, so you do not need to add the sauce. You can serve the meatballs with lettuce salad with broccoli. You may require 15-20 minutes to prepare the recipe.

Ingredients

- Beef- 0.9 lb
- Spanish chorizo- 1/3
- Egg- 1
- Almond flour- ½ cup
- Cumin- 1 tsp (ground)

- Paprika- 1 tsp

- Garlic- 2 cloves

- White onion- 1 small

- Oil or ghee- 1 tbsp

- Salt- to taste

- Cayenne pepper- to taste

Directions

- Take the white onion and dice them once peeled. Dice the garlic cloves and chorizo sausages as well.

- Take a pan and grease it with ghee or oil. Add onion, and then garlic. Cook for 30 seconds then adds chorizo. Cook for another 5-8 minutes. Cook the mixture until lightly crisped. Once crisped, set the mixture aside.

- Take a mixing bowl and add beef, one egg, paprika, salt, cayenne pepper, and cumin.

- Mix all the ingredients well and add already cooked chorizos, onion, and garlic in it.

- With the help of your hands, make medium-sized meatballs.

- Now heat the same pan where you cooked the chorizos. Once hot, add meatballs and let them cook for two to three minutes.

- Let the meatballs brown and change their side and cook for another 2 minutes. Then reduce the heat and cook the meatballs for other 6-9 minutes. Time can vary depending on the size of the meatballs.

- Remove and place the meatballs into a platter. You can freeze the meatballs as well.

2. Intermittent full English kebabs

If you do not like to buy readymade sausages, then this recipe is what you are seeking. You can make yourself sausages at home with our simple method. For kebabs, it only requires 10 minutes, but overall, it takes 30-35 minutes.

Ingredients

For homemade sausage meat

- Beef- 400 g (ground)

- Almond flour- ½ cup

- Sage- 1 tbsp

- Thyme- 1 tbsp

- Parsley- 1 tbsp

- Nutmeg- ¼ tsp

- White onion- 1 small (finely chopped)

- Fresh lemon juice- 1 tsp

- Dried marjoram- ½ tsp

- Salt- to taste

- Black pepper- to taste

- Dijon mustard- 1 tsp

For kebabs

- Homemade sausage meat

- White mushrooms 1 ½

- Cherry tomatoes- 1 cup

- Bacon- 6 slices

Directions

- Preheat oven at 200 °C/ 400 °F. Take all the herbs and wash them thoroughly. Chop them finely.

- Take a bowl and add meat, all herbs, white onion chopped, nutmeg, onion juice, and nutmeg.

- Then add mustard and mix all the ingredients well.

- With the help of your hands, make kebabs. Take bacon and wrap each kebab in the slice of bacon.

- Take skewers and start assembling the kebabs over them. Alternate the kebabs with tomatoes and mushrooms.

- Take out a baking tray and place the kebabs over baking paper.

- Place the kebabs into the oven for 25 minutes.

- Once cooked, remove the kebabs from oven and serve with fried eggs.

3. *Ribeye steak with Gremolata*

Everyone loves steak but being on a diet may prevent many to have the steak. The recipe encompasses the secure method to prepare juicy and delicious steak.

Ingredients

For steak:

- Ribeye steaks- 2 small

- Salt- to taste

- Black pepper- to taste

- Ghee- 1 tbsp

For Gremolata:

- Parsley leaves- 4 tbsp (freshly chopped)

- Garlic cloves- 2

- Lemon juice- 2 tsp

- Ghee- 3 tbsp

Directions

- Place steak at room temperature for 15 minutes. Remove excess of blood from the steak. Season it with salt and pepper. Add ghee. Season the steak with spices once you have tossed it with ghee or oil.

- Prepare Gremolata by adding parsley leaves and melted ghee. Add crushed garlic and lemon zest.

- Take a pan and add ghee in it fry for 2-3 minutes. Cook each side for 2 to 3 minutes and see when the steak becomes brown flip it to another side — Cook for 11 minutes.

- Once cooked, remove the steak from the pan and let it rest for 6 minutes. The best tip is to fold the steak in paper to make it rest properly.

- Then place on serving plate and serve with Gremolata.

Intermittent fasting smoothie recipes

Smoothies are often the favorites of many, and they are easy and quick to prepare. Here are the smoothies which provide you with delicious taste and are friendly for your diet.

1. Chocolate smoothie

This smoothie recipe encompasses eggs, but one can use 1-2 tbsp chia seeds as well. Or you can use one tbsp of coconut or almond butter. Instead of protein powder, one can use collagen or egg white. The time required for the preparation of the recipe is 5 minutes.

Ingredients

- Eggs- 2 large

- Coconut milk or heavy cream- 1 cup

- Protein powder- ¼ cup

- MCT oil or coconut oil- 1 tbsp

- Cacao powder- 1 tbsp

- Stevia extract- 3 to 5 drops

- Ice cubes & water- ¼ cup

- Cinnamon- ½ tsp

Directions

- Take the blender and add eggs into it. Add cream, cacao, stevia, ice, and heavy cream as well. Use chocolate stevia extract.

- Then add MCT oil or coconut oil (depending on your choice). Blend all the ingredients well. Make sure that you mix it well.

- You can also use cherry, almond, or orange pair in your chocolate smoothie.

- Blend until smooth and then serve chilled.

2. *Vanilla smoothie*

Smoothies are the choice of many, especially in the breakfasts. Smoothies require very little time for their preparation. You don't need to have any specific cooking skills for making smoothies. Just know the ingredients for your favorite smoothie and start making it. This recipe hardly takes 5 minutes for its preparation.

Ingredients

- Eggs- 2 (large size)

- Coconut milk or sour cream- ½ cup

- Vanilla or collagen powder- ¼ cup

- MCT oil or extra virgin coconut oil- 1 tbsp

- One vanilla bean or 1 tsp vanilla extract

- Stevia extract- 3 to 5 drops

- Water- ¼ cup

- Ice cubes- few

Note: if you are allergic to raw eggs then you can go for pasteurized eggs. To pasteurize eggs at your place, pour water in a saucepan and heat it. Place the eggs in it. Keep the eggs in the water for 2- 3 minutes. After 3 minutes, take out the eggs. Three minutes are enough to kill all the bacteria in the egg.

Directions

- Take the blender and put sour cream, protein powder, and water into it.

- You can use either vanilla beans or the vanilla extract. If you are using vanilla beans, you need to cut grains and take out the tiny seeds. If you don't like egg white, then you can go for protein powder or collagen powder.

- Now add the eggs. Then add stevia. If you still worry about using raw eggs, then you can use chia seeds.

- Now add ice. And MCT oil drops. If you don't have MCT oil or you don't like it then go for coconut oil.

- Blend until smooth and then serve chilled and delicious smoothie.

3. *Chocolate cheesecake smoothie*

Raspberries and chocolate are a favorite of many and are the perfect combination for a smoothie.

Ingredients

- Full-fat cream cheese- ¼ cup

- Heavy whipped cream- ¼ cup

- Raspberries- 1/3 cup

- Cacao powder- 1 tbsp

- Water- ½ cup

- MCT oil- 1 tbsp

Directions

- Take the blender and put dense whipped cream cheese, cacao powder, raspberries, MCT oil, and water.

- If you want then add a few drops of stevia.

- Blend it well until smooth. Pour ice cubes and blend further.

- Pour it in the glass and serve chilled.

Intermittent fasting snacks recipes

Intermittent Salmon BLT sandwich

Ingredients

- Bun- 1

- Salmon fillet- 1

- Avocado oil- 1 tbsp

- Bacon- 2 slices

- Lettuce leaves- 2

- Tomato slices- 1

- Red onion- 1 slice

- Mayonnaise- 1 tbsp

Directions

- Take the grill pan and heat it. Take salmon and season it with salt and pepper. Add oil to the pan and crisp your bacon.

- Cook each side of salmon for 5 minutes. Flip after 5 minutes. Remove the salmon.

- Slice the bun from half and start layering with lettuce leaves, tomatoes, onion, bacon, and mayonnaise.

- Then place salmon. Enjoy!

2. Intermittent McMuffins

Ingredients

For muffins

- Almond flour- ¼ cup

- Flaxmeal- ¼ cup

- Baking soda- ¼ tsp

- Egg- 1 large

- Heavy whipping cream- 2 tbsp

- Water- 2 tbsp

- Cheddar cheese- ¼ cup

- Salt- to taste

For filling

- Eggs- 2 large

- Ghee- 1 tbsp

- Butter- 1 tbsp

- Cheddar cheese- 2 slices

- Dijon mustard- 1 tsp

Directions

- Take a bowl and place all the ingredients in it. Add the eggs in it. Mix water and heavy cream. With the help of spoon mix all the ingredients thoroughly.

- Now add the cheese and combine well.

- Microwave for one minute.

- Take a pan, fry the egg in oil. Try to use muffin shaped pans to shape them just like muffins.

- Cut the already made muffins in half and spread butter on them. Now layer the cheese, eggs, and mustard over it. You can add lettuce leaves, spinach or chard if you want to. Enjoy!

Chapter 5: Good and Bad lessons from five years of Intermittent Fasting Diet

"Skipping breakfast isn't healthy, and I don't want to starve myself for twelve hours. Portion control is a better option because having six meals a day in smaller portions is the best way to control your diet." These were my words when my nutritionist suggested me to go for a three-month intermittent fasting schedule. I was there to consult her because I was going through a hell lot of issues including fatigue, lack of concentration, and habit of eating junk food. I also wanted to lose my weight to adopt a healthy lifestyle.

My nutritionist was insisting that intermittent fasting could solve all of my problems, but I was not ready to believe in that miracle.

After a long lecture from my doctor, I finally decided to give it a try because I was already fed up of different diet plans. I went to a gym on the last day of my intermittent fasting plan to check the progress

I had made. I was surprised to see a ten k.g reduction in my weight. This was something incredible for me because I didn't have any expectations from this diet schedule. So, I never checked my weight during the three months of the intermittent diet.

This result was enough to motivate me to go for another three months of intermittent fasting. Those three months were converted into two years and then five years of intermittent fasting. Now, after five years, I can say that choosing intermittent fasting was the most significant decision of my life. I am going to share with you whatever I experienced during this time so you may have a look at the aspects of intermittent fasting, which are usually not highlighted.

Intermittent diet is a lifestyle

Most people mix up the starvation without any thought with the intermittent fasting. But this is not at all true. Intermittent fasting is a habit or schedule of eating, which eventually becomes your lifestyle, which you can follow throughout your life. You must keep a record of your progress after intermittent fasting becomes your lifestyle. I used a few gadgets to track my development while fasting.

I used a mobile application called FatSecret to keep an eye on my daily calories intake. This app trained me to learn the number of calories different food items could provide me. After some time, I was able to guess the number of calories present in a food item by only having a look at it.

I used a scale to keep a check on my weight loss journey every week. The thing I learned from my experience is that weigh yourself at the same time every time of the day; otherwise, the results may vary.

Along with scale, I used a measuring tape to see if I had reduced inches also.

Your best friend during the intermittent fasting is water. Always carry a liter water bottle to keep yourself hydrated and to kick away the hunger pangs.

Your body is your expert

Usually, people are confused about what to eat during intermittent fasting. Selecting the most appropriate type of exercise according to your body's requirements is also very difficult. My experience says, "Always pay attention to how your body reacts to different foods and exercise schedule." Have a closer look at how your body reacts after consuming different foods. For example, if carbohydrate and fat-rich foods make you lazy, try vegetables or protein foods. Keep trying unless you get the most suitable option. Even after that, keep giving variation to your meals, so you don't feel bored with your monotonous routine diet.

Same goes for the exercise. Your body knows better which level and type of exercise suits it the best.

Keep the expectation level logical

In every diet plan, there are different phases. You may achieve the results quickly or slowly depends on various factors. The most crucial point is that every healthy diet plan takes a long time to affect but has lifetime results.

I lost almost all of my extra weight during the first year of intermittent fasting. The leaner me was super excited to have such beautiful results in only a year. But, the effects of my intermittent fasting slowed down soon. Then I realized that your body loses only unhealthy fat but keeps your muscle mass intact if you follow the right diet schedule.

Pair fasting with exercise to do miracles

If your goal of intermittent fasting is to become healthier, combine it with high-intensity exercise. The results will be far better as it happened in my case. Select any activity which suits your body like jogging, sprinting, swimming or even weight training. Try the high-intensity exercise in the fasted state, and the results will be even better and quicker.

The improvement in discipline and productivity

I felt more disciplined and productive during my intermittent fasting days. I could accomplish more tasks until afternoon than I used to do after having breakfast. The quality of work also improved because I was more focused while during the fasting days. But this energy level sustained until I would break my fast. The first meal after breaking my fast would make me feel lazy and unfocused.

You can get the best out of your productivity by scheduling your top priority work during the peak hours of your energy. It used to be before 2 pm in my case.

The discipline I learned from controlling my eating trained me for a lifetime. The improved will power as a result of the intermittent diet helped me to be stronger in the other aspects of my life also.

The reduction of discipline and productivity

Intermittent fasting can have adverse effects on your subject, productivity, and focus. This is very much true for the people who have lower hunger tolerance or have just started fasting. Hunger during fasting may cause mood swings and irritation, which affects your productivity. Low blood pressure and sugar level due to appetite decrease your focus and discipline. But don't give up. After a while, your body will learn to survive on stomach grumbling.

The best way to cope up with such situations is to pay attention to your body.be flexible and wait for your body to get accustomed to fasting.

Be consistent so that your body could adjust to the intermittent fasting routine quickly. Set a time for breaking the fast and follow it religiously. This step is crucial because too short fast cannot provide you with the benefits you expect from fasting. Similarly, too long fasting can cause health issues and demotivation.

Unhealthy intake during fasting

Intermittent fasting could lead you to eat unhealthily or junk food. You need firm control over your nerves to avoid junk food after breaking fast. But, if you consume unhealthy foods or empty calories, the goals of intermittent fasting can never be achieved. Avoid too sugary items while breaking fast because they suddenly raise the blood sugar level.

Enjoy life to the fullest

The best lesson I learned from my five years-long experience of intermittent fasting is that enjoy your life without worrying about achieving your fitness goals. I missed some unique dining experience only because I didn't want to disturb my eating routine. I was considering myself better than those people who could risk their healthy eating just for the sake of a delicious meal. But later, I realized that being fit, active, and healthy is only an essential part of life, not the entire life itself. Your mind and body need a break from the routine prohibitions sometimes. Let yourself enjoy the colors of life by enjoying a tasty breakfast or a full of fat hot dog once a while. This occasional cheating would give you motivation to pursue your eating schedule even more enthusiastically.

Conclusion

Intermittent fasting is the best way to lose that bothering weight in the most natural way. Setting up a schedule is all you need, and of course, you need to follow it. Intermittent fasting has many forms and types that you can follow.

You can choose any type that suits you best. You can manage and hold the strings of your life through it. Is weight a bother to you? You can control it with your perfect diet schedule, even some keto diet plan in it. If not a diet, many other options are waiting for you for your consideration. You can opt water-consuming plans, yoga, exercising staying happy, mental stability, etc.

If you do not consider obesity as a problematic situation, you might end up piling yourself for the worst. There can be many greater problems waiting for you. Like diabetes etc. their stages might advance as well. You would end up spending tons to your doctor. Hence it is better to control it in the initial step. You can gain control over yourself, over your mind, over your decisions and how you want your body to operate. You need to control your diet. By that, it does not mean, you cannot eat what you want to. You certainly can. But you just need to know the timings that you are allowed to dine in.

The diseases that can cling to your body can destroy your life. Their life expectancy rate can also be endangered. Women are also persistent in consuming fatty foods full of cholesterol, high fructose levels, high sugar levels, syrups, and trans fats even.

Researchers showed that women find it even more challenging to maintain a schedule than dieting. Hence, they are unable to stick to a gym routine. However, they can stick to intermittent fasting because it has certain types that are very easy to follow and stick with.

You can say goodbye to your obesity and see the difference in just a month. It is very helpful for you if you are lazy and tired of going to the gym. Stick to the plan by only being seated and watching a movie. No need for dieting obviously. You need your essential proteins, but you need them at their time when your body requires for it. You need to follow your body's needs rather than the love of your taste buds asking for creamy pulps all the time.